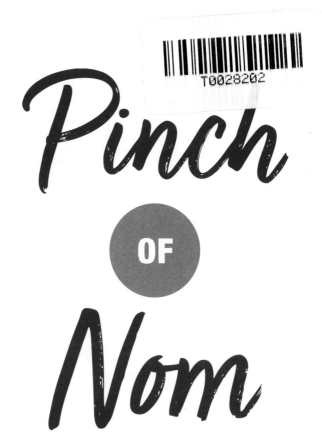

Pinch

OF

Nom

FAMILY MEAL
PLANNER

Pinch

OF

Nom

FAMILY MEAL PLANNER

Includes 26 Recipes

bluebird
books for life

First published 2022 by Bluebird
an imprint of Pan Macmillan
The Smithson, 6 Briset Street, London EC1M 5NR

EU representative: Macmillan Publishers Ireland Ltd, 1st Floor,
The Liffey Trust Centre, 117–126 Sheriff Street Upper Dublin 1, D01 YC43

Associated companies throughout the world
www.panmacmillan.com

ISBN 978-1-5290-7946-3

1 3 5 7 9 8 6 4 2

A CIP catalogue record for this book is available from the British Library.

Printed and bound in China.

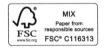

Publisher Carole Tonkinson
Managing Editor Martha Burley
Senior Production Controller Sarah Badhan
Art Direction, Design and Illustration Emma Wells, Studio Nic&Lou
Additional illustrations Shutterstock

Visit www.panmacmillan.com/bluebird to read more about all our books
and to buy them. You will also find features, author interviews and
news of any author events, and you can sign up for e-newsletters
so that you're always first to hear about our new releases.

CONTENTS

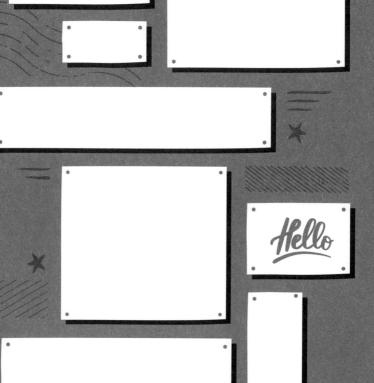

Use this page to scribble down page numbers from the planner – so you can easily refer to a particular week or day of progress, or a recipe you love.

Hello

WELCOME TO THE
Food Planner

When it comes to family mealtimes, we know how important it is to get ahead and feel organised. We designed this handy planner to give you space to plan tasty, crowd-pleasing meals for you and your family, and keep track of what you've all enjoyed each day. At a glance you can see your meal choices for previous days, and what you've planned for the weeks ahead. Thanks to recipes, shopping lists and batch-cooking guidance, this planner is the perfect tool to highlight your family favourites, save time and cook delicious Pinch of Nom meals.

We've kept this 3-month planner nice and compact so that it's easy to carry with you. We know it's more convenient to fill in your food on our planners as you go, especially when you're busy and out and about most of the day. We've also included hearty, comforting, satisfying recipes that all the family will love.

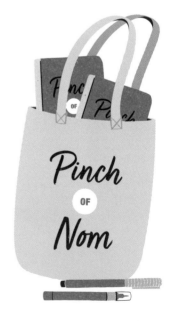

NOTE: *While this planner is designed to help out with organising meals for the whole family, the weight-tracking features are intended for individual use and for the adults of the household only.*

ABOUT
Pinch OF Nom

Just a few years ago, Kay and Kate started Pinch of Nom to share their slimming recipes with a select few friends and family. Fast forward to today and Pinch of Nom has become a phenomenon, with four best-selling cookbooks available in more than 20 countries and translated into 16 languages!

What started as a small idea has grown into a combined Facebook community of over 2 million supportive and friendly members, centred around delicious recipes. Guided by conversations with our incredible community, we wanted this planner to be about sharing and enjoying healthy family favourites one week at a time.

UPDATED
Features

This planner is all about helping you to stay organised and on track. You'll find convenient pull-out shopping lists and a full recipe index in the back. This is our most family-friendly planner to date, so we've included extra tips about batch cooking and provided areas to jot down what you have in the freezer and what foods need using up, helping you prevent wasting food and unnecessary costs!

We also know that so many of you are following meal plans or tracking calories and values. So just like our other planners, inside this book there are places for the adults in the family to track their slimming progress and make healthy eating so much more achievable.

With 26 brand-new and exclusive recipes, you can try two new dishes a week as part of your meal plan. And it's fun to celebrate every little success with some cute and colourful NOM-tastic stickers, too.

How to
USE THE PLANNER

This planner is your new go-to companion for creating family-friendly meals that'll help you keep on top of your cooking and shopping. With seven-day meal planners to prepare for the coming week, pull-out shopping lists, and space to record what's going into the freezer or needs using up, it helps you to streamline your daily routine. It's a handy space to log your meal ideas, with inspiring, delicious recipes that'll encourage your family to gather around the table.

Carry this portable journal with you when you're out and about so you've always got a place to jot down some inspiration for next week's meals. It's important to remember that this food planner is a blank canvas for you to use as you wish. Not only can you plan your meals, but you can also take a moment to think about how you're feeling and any achievements. Do you have any positive or negative reflections from the previous week? Perhaps a day that was full of your favourite recipes? Although it sounds simple, we believe a mindful approach to organisation will make a big difference each week!

For the adults in the family on any kind of slimming journey, we understand how hard it can be to stay on track. This planner helps to make it simple to feed your family AND, if you wish, it also gives you the tools to hit your slimming target.

We also know, from first-hand experience, that support and encouragement is vital when you are balancing family life. We've incorporated the PON community, and support offered by our online community, by including some motivational thoughts and phrases for a burst of focus and inspiration throughout this planner.

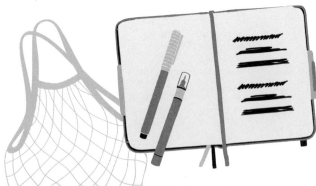

The
RECIPES

We love to bring you recipes that show that healthy food doesn't have to be boring food.

All of the recipes in this planner are hearty, filling family favourites. They are the perfect accompaniment to our *Comfort Food* cookbook, helping you plan a week-by-week menu with crowd-pleasing dishes that are full of flavour. Each recipe falls into a category that is explained on the next page, which we hope will make food planning easier.

To keep the recipes accessible, we've featured simple ingredients that can be used time and again to help you save on cost. If you spot an ingredient that seems less common, then this means that we think it's worth including as it adds a really special touch to the dish. We love using versatile flavourings such as stocks and sauces in our recipes for big splashes of flavour. Stock pots, soy sauce, fish sauce and Worcestershire sauce are high in salt, so swap with reduced-salt varieties if you prefer.

These recipes are also incredibly versatile. You can also make switches to suit a range of diets, swap ingredients if you can't get hold of something, or throw in extra veg if it needs using up. Anything goes! Remember, you can always use up your extra veg and then batch cook most of these recipes to freeze for future ready-made meals in a flash.

Cooking should be fun and these recipes are perfect for getting the whole family involved. We know cooking together is quality time – especially when you can all gather around the table together to enjoy the food you love.

As always, we hope that you enjoy making these recipes as much as we loved developing them for you.

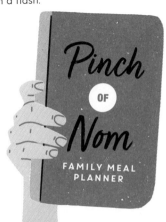

Recipe Categories

EVERYDAY LIGHT

Cook these recipes freely throughout the week. All the meals in this category are under 400 calories per serving (including accompaniments, unless they are optional) and all sides, snacks and sweet treats under 200 calories. Keep an eye on the values if you are counting calories, but these recipes should make it easy to stay under your allowance.

WEEKLY INDULGENCE

These recipes are still low in calories, at between 400 and 500 calories, or 200–300 for sides, snacks and sweet treats, but they should be saved for once or twice a week for adults who are looking to slim. Mix them into your meal plans alongside Everyday Light recipes for variety.

SPECIAL OCCASION

These recipes are often lower in calories than their full-fat counterparts, but, for adult slimmers, they need to be saved for a special occasion. This category indicates any main meals that are over 500 calories or over 300 for sides, snacks and sweet treats.

KCALS AND CARB VALUES

All of our recipes have been worked out as complete meals, using standardised portion sizes for any accompaniments as advised by the British Nutrition Foundation. Carb values are included for those who prefer to measure their intake.

GLUTEN-FREE RECIPES

We have marked gluten-free recipes with a GF icon. All these recipes are either free of gluten, or we have suggested gluten-free ingredient swaps of common ingredients, such as stock cubes and Worcestershire sauce. Please check labelling to ensure the product you buy is gluten free.

Calories and Values

The calorie counts provided have been worked out per individual serving for your convenience. Please remember that the calorie counts don't include optional side dishes or accompaniments such as potatoes or rice: these are serving suggestions only and can be swapped to whatever you prefer.

We haven't included 'values' from any mainstream diet programmes, as these can change quite often and we want this planner to be an up-to-date resource that you can use time and again.

Our Recipe Icons

V Suitable for vegetarians

VG Suitable for vegans

F Suitable for freezing (see freezing guidelines opposite)

BF Suitable for batch cooking

DF Suitable for those following a dairy-free diet

GF Suitable for those following a gluten-free diet

HOW TO
Batch Cook

Batch cooking and meal planning go hand in hand. Our incredible community loves getting organised with a good batch-cooking session, which is why we've included some of our top tips for batch cooking below and throughout this planner. Including some leftovers in your meal plan for busy days can be a life-saver. There's nothing more comforting than knowing you've got a portion of something delicious waiting for you in the fridge, and all you need to do is reheat it.

• **Why batch cook?** Making a bigger batch of a dish each time you cook can help to save time, money and prevent food waste too. It's a no-brainer!

• **When should I batch cook?** One of our top tips is to cook a couple of different dishes on a weekend, to store away for a quick win on a busier day. That way, you can enjoy your favourite recipes on the days when you get in late and don't fancy cooking for hours.

• **Is eating leftovers 'boring'?** You can change it up so it never feels like you're eating the same thing on repeat. Lots of recipes can be served with different side dishes or a variety of accompaniments to keep it interesting! Try serving a meal with rice one night and chips the next.

• **Divide up your portions** and allow to cool and freeze as quickly as possible. This means you don't have to refrigerate or freeze leftovers in bulk. There's nothing worse than chiselling away at a huge, frozen block of food! Individual portions also defrost a lot quicker.

• **Check you've got space** in your fridge or freezer before you start cooking!

• **Use airtight containers** or freezer bags. If you invest in some decent, microwave-safe containers, they won't crack or melt. Make sure they are properly sealed to avoid freezer burn (uninvited air damaging your food).

• **Use refrigerated leftovers for lunch or dinner** within 2 days. Many recipes like curries and chillies taste even better after 24 hours in the fridge, but they won't keep for much longer than that.

• **Label** your batch-cooked meals. Extra portions can be packaged up into freezer-safe containers and stored away for busier days, but be sure to write the date you made it (and what it is!) on a freezer-proof sticker. Meals can be frozen for 3–6 months, although they will taste better the sooner they're eaten.

• **Defrost food thoroughly** in the fridge or microwave before reheating it.

• **Reheat and eat food within 24 hours** of defrosting it. NHS guidelines (correct at the time of writing) state that you should reheat food until it reaches 90°C/158°F and holds that temperature for 2 minutes. Make sure it's piping hot throughout. Stir while reheating to ensure this.

• **Only ever reheat food once.**

One

CHANGE +/-   CURRENT WEIGHT

— *The Week Ahead* —————————————————

REMINDERS FOR THIS WEEK

LAST WEEK, THESE THINGS WENT WELL...

IN THE FREEZER   DATE   FOOD TO USE UP   DATE

CREAMY CHICKEN *and* LEMON NOODLE SOUP

🕐 **15 MINS** | 🍲 **35 MINS** | ✕ **SERVES 4**

Use GF stock cubes and pasta

Is it just us or is a bowl of chicken soup the definition of comfort food? This soup is simple to make and a great way to use up leftover cooked chicken breasts. To build up satisfying, cosy flavours, we've used lots of veggies, smooth cream cheese and an unexpected zesty lemon twist. The perfect pick-me-up if you're feeling under the weather!

PER SERVING
250 KCAL / 24G CARBS

low-calorie cooking spray
1 medium onion, peeled and finely chopped
2 carrots, peeled and finely diced
1 celery stick, finely diced
2 garlic cloves, peeled and crushed
1.4 litres chicken stock (2 chicken stock cubes dissolved in 1.4 litres boiling water)
juice of 1 lemon
100g low-fat cream cheese
300g cooked skinless chicken, shredded
75g dried linguine, broken into 3 pieces
handful of fresh basil leaves, shredded, plus extra to serve
100g frozen garden peas
30g spinach
sea salt and freshly ground black pepper

Everyday Light

Spray a saucepan with low-calorie cooking spray and place over a medium heat. Add the onion, carrots and celery and sauté for 5 minutes until beginning to soften. Add the garlic and cook for a further minute, then add the stock and simmer for 15 minutes.

Stir in the lemon juice and cream cheese until it has thoroughly melted, then add the shredded chicken and the linguine. Stir well and cook for 10 minutes.

Stir in the basil, peas and spinach and cook for another 2–3 minutes.

Taste and season with salt and pepper if you wish. Serve in bowls, garnished with a few basil leaves.

SWAP THIS: Substitute linguine for spaghetti if you prefer. Swap the fresh basil for 1 teaspoon of dried basil.

TIP: If you don't have any chicken leftovers, poach 2 small skinless breasts in water for 20 minutes, until cooked through. You can then use the poaching liquid to make the stock with the stock cubes.

Weekly Meal Planner

	BREAKFAST	LUNCH
MONDAY		
TUESDAY		
WEDNESDAY		
THURSDAY		
FRIDAY		
SATURDAY		
SUNDAY		

Weekly Meal Planner

DINNER	SNACK	NOTES

Day One

BREAKFAST	VALUES
TOTAL	

LUNCH	VALUES
TOTAL	

DINNER	VALUES
TOTAL	

SNACKS AND TREATS	VALUES
TOTAL	
DAILY TOTAL	

WATER

⬡ ⬡ ⬡ ⬡
⬡ ⬡ ⬡ ⬡

Notes

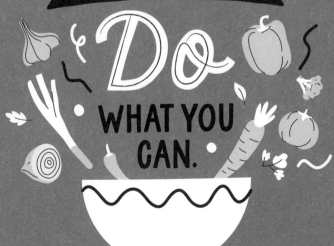

Start

WHERE YOU ARE.

Use

WHAT YOU HAVE.

Do

WHAT YOU CAN.

BREAKFAST QUESADILLA

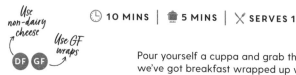

Use non-dairy cheese

Use GF wraps

DF **GF**

🕐 **10 MINS** | 🍲 **5 MINS** | ✕ **SERVES 1**

PER SERVING
382 KCAL / 24G CARBS

low-calorie cooking spray
1 smoked bacon medallion, diced
2 medium eggs
1 small low-calorie soft tortilla wrap (about 18cm/7in in diameter)
20g reduced-fat Cheddar, finely grated
3 cherry tomatoes, sliced
sea salt and freshly ground black pepper

TO ACCOMPANY *(optional)*
dollop of reduced sugar and salt tomato ketchup (+ 13 kcal) or reduced sugar and salt brown sauce (+ 20 kcal)

> **SWAP THIS:**
> We added sliced tomatoes to our quesadilla, but you could try adding other vegetables such as sliced button mushrooms or onions instead. You would need to fry them first with the bacon until all the juices have evaporated.

Pour yourself a cuppa and grab the frying pan – we've got breakfast wrapped up with this tasty Breakfast Quesadilla. With a mix of bacon, eggs, juicy tomatoes and melty cheese, this low-calorie tortilla quesadilla will leave you feeling full and satisfied until lunchtime. What you fill it with is up to you!

Everyday Light ———————————————

Spray a small non-stick frying pan with low-calorie cooking spray and place over a medium heat. When hot, add the diced bacon and fry for 1–2 minutes until cooked through. Transfer the bacon to a plate and set aside.

Crack the eggs into a small bowl, beat with a fork and season with salt and pepper.

Place the frying pan over a low-medium heat (there's no need to wash the pan first or spray it again with low-calorie cooking spray).

When the pan is hot, add the eggs and tilt the pan slightly so that the eggs swirl around to completely cover the bottom of the pan.

Cook gently for 1–2 minutes, without stirring, or until the eggs have set like a very thin omelette and are nearly cooked but are still wet on the surface.

While the egg mixture is still wet on the surface, place the tortilla wrap on top. Press the wrap down lightly with a fish slice so that it sticks to the egg.

Flip over the egg and wrap layer using a fish slice so that the egg is facing up. Scatter the bacon, cheese and tomato slices over the egg in an even layer, fold the quesadilla in half and cook for about 30 seconds or until golden on the underside.

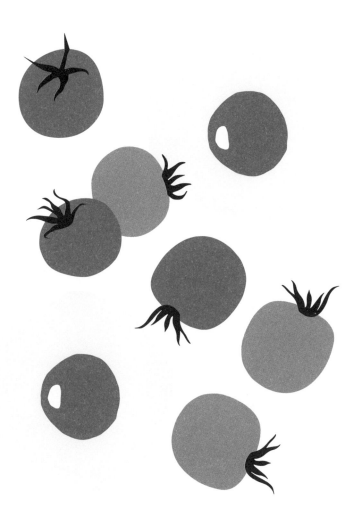

Flip over and cook on the other side for a further
30 seconds or until the cheese has melted and the
quesadilla is golden.

Cut in half and serve hot, either alone or with a
dollop of tomato ketchup or brown sauce.

Day Two

BREAKFAST	VALUES
TOTAL	

LUNCH	VALUES
TOTAL	

DINNER	VALUES
TOTAL	

SNACKS AND TREATS	VALUES
TOTAL	
DAILY TOTAL	

WATER

○ ○ ○ ○
○ ○ ○ ○

Notes

Day Three

BREAKFAST	VALUES
TOTAL	

LUNCH	VALUES
TOTAL	

DINNER	VALUES
TOTAL	

SNACKS AND TREATS	VALUES
TOTAL	
DAILY TOTAL	

WATER

○ ○ ○ ○
○ ○ ○ ○

Notes

Day Four

BREAKFAST	VALUES
TOTAL	

LUNCH	VALUES
TOTAL	

DINNER	VALUES
TOTAL	

SNACKS AND TREATS	VALUES
TOTAL	
DAILY TOTAL	

WATER

○ ○ ○ ○
○ ○ ○ ○

Notes

Day Five

BREAKFAST	VALUES
TOTAL	

LUNCH	VALUES
TOTAL	

DINNER	VALUES
TOTAL	

SNACKS AND TREATS	VALUES
TOTAL	
DAILY TOTAL	

WATER

○ ○ ○ ○
○ ○ ○ ○

'I am absolutely loving this planner.' **RACHEL**

Day Six

BREAKFAST	VALUES
TOTAL	

LUNCH	VALUES
TOTAL	

DINNER	VALUES
TOTAL	

SNACKS AND TREATS	VALUES
TOTAL	
DAILY TOTAL	

WATER

○ ○ ○ ○
○ ○ ○ ○

Notes

Day Seven

BREAKFAST	VALUES
TOTAL	

LUNCH	VALUES
TOTAL	

DINNER	VALUES
TOTAL	

SNACKS AND TREATS	VALUES
TOTAL	
DAILY TOTAL	

WATER

○ ○ ○ ○
○ ○ ○ ○

Notes _____

_____

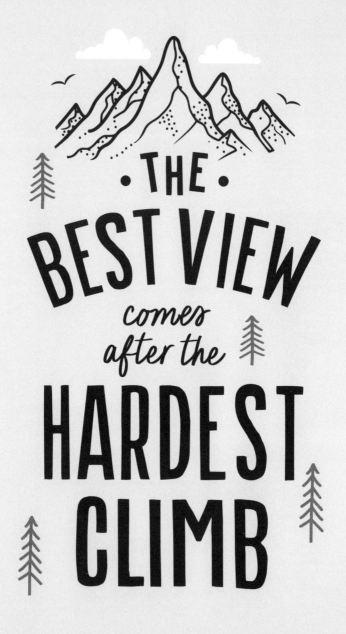

THE BEST VIEW comes after the HARDEST CLIMB

Shopping List 1

....
....
....
....
....
....
....
....
....
....
....
....
....
....
....
....
....
....
....
....

Shopping List 2

....
....
....
....
....
....
....
....
....
....
....
....
....
....
....
....
....
....
....
....

Shopping List 1

....
....
....
....
....
....
....
....
....
....
....
....
....
....
....
....
....
....

Shopping List 2

....
....
....
....
....
....
....
....
....
....
....
....
....
....
....
....
....
....

Two

CHANGE +/-   CURRENT WEIGHT

— *The Week Ahead* —————————————

REMINDERS FOR THIS WEEK

LAST WEEK, THESE THINGS WENT WELL...

IN THE FREEZER   DATE   FOOD TO USE UP   DATE

Weekly Meal Planner

	BREAKFAST	LUNCH
MONDAY		
TUESDAY		
WEDNESDAY		
THURSDAY		
FRIDAY		
SATURDAY		
SUNDAY		

Weekly Meal Planner

DINNER	SNACK	NOTES

KORMA LAMB CHOPS

⏱ **10 MINS** | 🍲 **25 MINS** | ✕ **SERVES 2**

PER SERVING
372 KCAL / 5.1G CARBS

low-calorie cooking spray
4 lamb cutlets, trimmed of
    excess fat
½ medium onion, peeled
    and finely diced
1 garlic clove, peeled and
    crushed
1.5cm (¾in) piece of
    root ginger, peeled and
    finely grated
2 tsp mild curry powder
2 tsp tomato puree
250ml coconut dairy-free
    milk alternative
1 tsp lemon juice
15g ground almonds
1 tsp mango chutney
sea salt and freshly ground
    black pepper
small handful of fresh
    coriander, roughly
    chopped, to serve

TO ACCOMPANY *(optional)*
50g raw basmati rice per
    portion, cooked
    according to packet
    instructions
    (+ 173 kcal per 125g
    cooked serving)

These delicious lamb chops simmered in a fragrant, creamy korma sauce are perfect comfort food. This might not be a traditional combination, but lamb always tastes incredible when it's served with a sweet sauce (think redcurrant gravy or mint sauce). Our dairy-free, low-calorie korma is just sweet enough, with almonds and a hint of juicy mango to complement the lamb flavours.

Everyday Light ─────────────────

Spray a deep, non-stick frying pan with low-calorie cooking spray and place over a high heat. Season the lamb cutlets with a little salt and pepper then, when the pan is hot, place the cutlets in the pan and sear on each side for about a minute until well browned. Remove from the pan and set to one side.

Allow the pan to cool a little, and if there are any black bits in the pan wipe them out with some kitchen roll as this will discolour your sauce. Reduce the heat to medium and give the pan another spray with low-calorie cooking spray. Add the onion and sauté for 5 minutes, until soft, then add the garlic, ginger and curry powder and cook for another minute until fragrant. Add the tomato puree, coconut dairy-free milk alternative, lemon juice, ground almonds and mango chutney and stir well.

Return the chops to the pan and bring to a simmer. When bubbling, cover with a lid, reduce the heat and cook for 10 minutes.

After 10 minutes, turn the chops over and continue cooking, uncovered, for another 5 minutes.

Taste the sauce and season with a little salt if you think it needs it. Sprinkle over the chopped coriander and serve.

WEEK 2

Day One

BREAKFAST	VALUES
TOTAL	

LUNCH	VALUES
TOTAL	

DINNER	VALUES
TOTAL	

SNACKS AND TREATS	VALUES
TOTAL	
DAILY TOTAL	

WATER

◇ ◇ ◇ ◇
◇ ◇ ◇ ◇

Meal of the Day

Day Two

BREAKFAST	VALUES
TOTAL	

LUNCH	VALUES
TOTAL	

DINNER	VALUES
TOTAL	

SNACKS AND TREATS	VALUES
TOTAL	
DAILY TOTAL	

WATER

Notes

Day Three

BREAKFAST	VALUES
TOTAL	

LUNCH	VALUES
TOTAL	

DINNER	VALUES
TOTAL	

SNACKS AND TREATS	VALUES
TOTAL	
DAILY TOTAL	

WATER

◇ ◇ ◇ ◇
◇ ◇ ◇ ◇

Notes

CHILLI MEATLOAF

Use GF breadcrumbs and Henderson's relish ←

🕐 **1 HOUR 20 MINS** | 🍲 **20 MINS** | ✕ **SERVES 6**

PER SERVING
235 KCAL / 19G CARBS

SPECIAL EQUIPMENT
900g (2lb) loaf tin

low-calorie cooking spray
1 medium onion, peeled
 and very finely chopped
2 mixed peppers, deseeded
 and very finely chopped
500g extra-lean minced
 beef
1 x 400g tin kidney beans,
 drained, rinsed and
 roughly mashed with
 a fork
1½ tsp garlic granules
1 tsp ground cumin
2 tsp mild chilli powder (or
 use hot if you prefer)
1 tsp dried oregano
1½ tbsp tomato puree
1 tbsp Henderson's relish or
 Worcestershire sauce
40g panko breadcrumbs
1 medium egg, beaten
small handful of fresh
 coriander, chopped
sea salt and freshly ground
 black pepper

Inspired by Mexican flavours, we've added mild chilli spices and a sweet, tangy glaze to this family-sized meatloaf recipe. Our mixture goes a long way as it's packed with tasty veggies and beans, making it budget friendly as well as low in calories. Better yet, every slice stays moist and delicious (even after it has been frozen!), so it's a super easy batch-cook option.

Everyday Light ————————————

Preheat the oven to 180°C (fan 160°C/gas mark 4). Spray the loaf tin with low-calorie cooking spray. Cut a strip of greaseproof paper or baking parchment the same width as your tin and twice as long. Line the bottom and up the two ends. This will make it easier to remove the meatloaf.

Spray a frying pan with low-calorie cooking spray and place over a medium heat. Add the onions and peppers and fry for 6–8 minutes until softened. Allow to cool slightly.

Place the onions and peppers in a large mixing bowl and mix with the remaining meatloaf ingredients until well combined. You can check the seasoning by frying penny-sized pieces of the mixture in the frying pan until cooked, tasting and adjusting the seasoning accordingly.

Press the meatloaf mixture firmly into the greased and lined loaf tin, pop on a baking sheet, and bake in the oven for 50 minutes. Meanwhile, mix the glaze ingredients together in a small bowl.

After 50 minutes, remove the meatloaf from the oven and brush over the glaze. Return to the oven for a further 20 minutes.

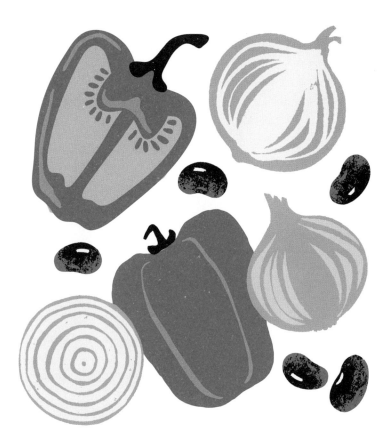

FOR THE GLAZE
2 tbsp tomato ketchup
½ tsp granulated
  sweetener or caster
  sugar
¼ tsp garlic granules
¼ tsp mild chilli powder
  (optional)

TO ACCOMPANY *(optional)*
80g steamed green
  vegetables (+ 35 kcal
  per serving)

Leave the meatloaf to rest in the tin for 15 minutes, before loosening the edges with a knife and lifting it out of the tin.

Carefully slice into six pieces and serve.

TIP: A probe thermometer is a great way to ensure this meatloaf is thoroughly cooked without having to cut into it. You need to achieve a temperature of 75°C in the middle of the meatloaf. If you don't have a loaf tin, firmly press the mix into a loaf shape with your hands, place on a baking tray, and cook as instructed above.

Day Four

BREAKFAST	VALUES
TOTAL	

LUNCH	VALUES
TOTAL	

DINNER	VALUES
TOTAL	

SNACKS AND TREATS	VALUES
TOTAL	
DAILY TOTAL	

WATER

○ ○ ○ ○
○ ○ ○ ○

> *'I went through all my books and planner marking out recipes I want to try.'* **JOANNE**

Day Five

BREAKFAST	VALUES
TOTAL	

LUNCH	VALUES
TOTAL	

DINNER	VALUES
TOTAL	

SNACKS AND TREATS	VALUES
TOTAL	
DAILY TOTAL	

WATER

Notes

Day Six

BREAKFAST	VALUES
TOTAL	

LUNCH	VALUES
TOTAL	

DINNER	VALUES
TOTAL	

SNACKS AND TREATS	VALUES
TOTAL	
DAILY TOTAL	

WATER

○ ○ ○ ○
○ ○ ○ ○

Notes

Day Seven

BREAKFAST	VALUES
TOTAL	

LUNCH	VALUES
TOTAL	

DINNER	VALUES
TOTAL	

SNACKS AND TREATS	VALUES
TOTAL	
DAILY TOTAL	

WATER

○ ○ ○ ○
○ ○ ○ ○

Notes

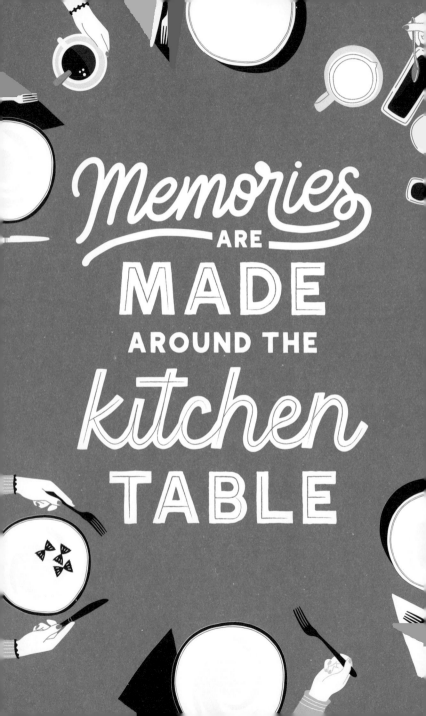

Three

CHANGE +/-   CURRENT WEIGHT

— The Week Ahead —————————

REMINDERS FOR THIS WEEK

LAST WEEK, THESE THINGS WENT WELL...

IN THE FREEZER   DATE   **FOOD TO USE UP**   DATE

Weekly Meal Planner

	BREAKFAST	LUNCH
MONDAY		
TUESDAY		
WEDNESDAY		
THURSDAY		
FRIDAY		
SATURDAY		
SUNDAY		

Weekly Meal Planner

DINNER	SNACK	NOTES

Day One

BREAKFAST	VALUES
TOTAL	

LUNCH	VALUES
TOTAL	

DINNER	VALUES
TOTAL	

SNACKS AND TREATS	VALUES
TOTAL	
DAILY TOTAL	

WATER

Notes

Day Two

BREAKFAST	VALUES
TOTAL	

LUNCH	VALUES
TOTAL	

DINNER	VALUES
TOTAL	

SNACKS AND TREATS	VALUES
TOTAL	
DAILY TOTAL	

WATER

Notes

JALAPEÑO POPPER SAUSAGE ROLLS

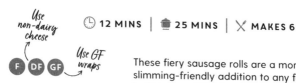

Use non-dairy cheese

Use GF wraps

F **DF** **GF**

⏱ **12 MINS** | 🍲 **25 MINS** | ✕ **MAKES 6**

PER SERVING
166 KCAL / 12G CARBS

300g 5%-fat minced pork
½ small onion, peeled and finely diced
40g jalapeños in brine, drained and finely diced
¼ tsp garlic granules
¼ tsp English mustard powder
¼ tsp dried parsley
3 string cheese, cut in half
low-calorie cooking spray
3 low-calorie soft tortilla wraps
1 medium egg, beaten
sea salt and freshly ground black pepper

These fiery sausage rolls are a moreish yet slimming-friendly addition to any family picnic or buffet spread! While a traditional jalapeño popper comes deep-fried in breadcrumbs and stuffed with cheese, we've encased a cheesy blend of meat, mustard and jalapeños in a low-calorie tortilla wrap. Bake until crisp and pull them apart for satisfying, gooey goodness!

Everyday Light ———————————

Preheat the oven to 220°C (fan 200°C/gas mark 7). Spray a baking tray with low-calorie cooking spray.

Put the minced pork in a mixing bowl along with the onion, jalapeños, garlic granules, mustard powder and parsley and season with salt and pepper. Mix thoroughly until fully combined. Divide the meat mixture evenly into six pieces. Flatten a piece slightly in your hand and add half a string cheese to the centre. Wrap the meat mixture around the cheese and shape into a sausage shape. Repeat with the remaining mince mixture and string cheese to make another five.

Place the sausages on the baking tray and cook in the oven for 15 minutes.

Remove them from the oven and leave them to cool until they are cool enough to handle.

Lay a wrap flat on the work surface and brush the wrap all over with beaten egg. Place two sausages horizontally end to end along the edge of the wrap. Roll up tightly, making sure you finish with the seam underneath, then cut in half.

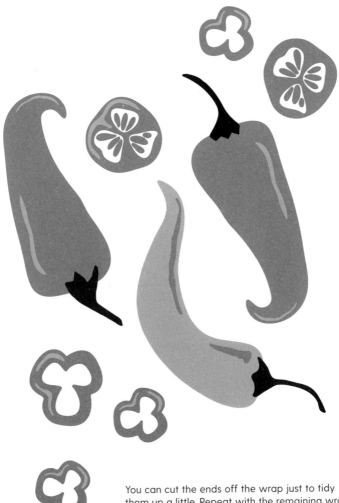

You can cut the ends off the wrap just to tidy them up a little. Repeat with the remaining wraps and sausage mixture.

Place the six sausage rolls seam side down on the baking tray and brush each one with the remaining beaten egg. Cook in the oven for another 10 minutes, or until they are crisp and golden brown. Serve.

Day Three

BREAKFAST	VALUES
TOTAL	

LUNCH	VALUES
TOTAL	

DINNER	VALUES
TOTAL	

SNACKS AND TREATS	VALUES
TOTAL	
DAILY TOTAL	

WATER

$\lozenge$ $\lozenge$ $\lozenge$ $\lozenge$

$\lozenge$ $\lozenge$ $\lozenge$ $\lozenge$

Notes

Day Four

BREAKFAST	VALUES
TOTAL	

LUNCH	VALUES
TOTAL	

DINNER	VALUES
TOTAL	

SNACKS AND TREATS	VALUES
TOTAL	
DAILY TOTAL	

WATER

○ ○ ○ ○

○ ○ ○ ○

Notes

Day Five

BREAKFAST	VALUES
TOTAL	

LUNCH	VALUES
TOTAL	

DINNER	VALUES
TOTAL	

SNACKS AND TREATS	VALUES
TOTAL	
DAILY TOTAL	

WATER

○ ○ ○ ○
○ ○ ○ ○

Notes

WEEK 3

Day Six

BREAKFAST	VALUES
TOTAL	

LUNCH	VALUES
TOTAL	

DINNER	VALUES
TOTAL	

SNACKS AND TREATS	VALUES
TOTAL	
DAILY TOTAL	

WATER

○ ○ ○ ○
○ ○ ○ ○

'Loving the latest Pinch of Nom planner, full of fabulousness to keep you motivated.' **ZOE**

FISH *and* CHIP WRAP

Cooked fish
and chips
only →

Use DF
tartare
sauce →

(F) (DF) (GF)

Use GF
breadcrumbs,
wraps and
→ tartare sauce

🕐 **10 MINS** | 🍲 **25 MINS** | ✕ **SERVES 4**

PER SERVING
272 KCAL / 37G CARBS

1 medium slice of brown
  bread, made into
  breadcrumbs (around
  37g) – see page 75
1 medium egg, beaten
low-calorie cooking spray
120g skinless, boneless cod
  or haddock fillet, cut into
  4 pieces
1 floury potato (about 136g),
  such as Maris Piper or
  King Edward peeled
  and cut into 1cm
  (½in)-wide chips
sea salt and freshly ground
  black pepper

TO SERVE
120g tinned mushy peas
4 low-calorie soft tortilla
  wraps
8 tsp tartare sauce (2 tsp
  per wrap)
20g rocket leaves

Anyone fancy fish and chips for lunch? This recipe
has all the elements of your favourite chippy order,
wrapped up in a soft, low-calorie tortilla. We've even
included the mushy peas! It feels like such a treat for
lunch, and you can always serve it with a few extra
chips for a really satisfying midweek dinner.

Everyday Light

Preheat the oven to 210°C (fan 190°C/gas mark 6).

Put the breadcrumbs on a plate and season with salt
and pepper. Put the beaten egg in a shallow bowl.
Spray a baking tray with low-calorie cooking spray.
Dip the pieces of fish one at a time into the beaten
egg, and then coat with the breadcrumbs. Place the
breadcrumbed fish on the baking tray and spray each
piece with low-calorie cooking spray. Add the potato
chips to the baking tray with the breadcrumbed fish
and spray with low-calorie cooking spray, then bake
in the oven for 25 minutes, turning everything midway
through, until the fish pieces and the chips are golden
and cooked through.

Gently heat the mushy peas in a small saucepan or
in the microwave until piping hot.

To assemble the wraps: Lay a tortilla wrap flat on
the work surface and cut it halfway up the middle.
Imagine the tortilla is split into four sections. Spread
1 teaspoon of the tartare sauce onto the bottom left
quarter and place a fish piece and some chips onto
the top left quarter. Add mushy peas to the top right
quarter and spread another teaspoon of the tartare
sauce onto the bottom right quarter and pile on the
rocket. Fold the bottom left quarter up over the top
left quarter, then fold that over onto the top right
quarter, then fold over onto the bottom right quarter.
You should have a folded triangle shape with your
filling inside. Repeat to make the other three wraps.

MAKE YOURSELF A PRIORITY

Day Seven

BREAKFAST	VALUES
TOTAL	

LUNCH	VALUES
TOTAL	

DINNER	VALUES
TOTAL	

SNACKS AND TREATS	VALUES
TOTAL	
DAILY TOTAL	

WATER

Notes

Shopping List 1

....
....
....
....
....
....
....
....
....
....
....
....
....
....
....
....
....
....
....
....

Shopping List 2

....
....
....
....
....
....
....
....
....
....
....
....
....
....
....
....
....
....
....

Shopping List ①

....
....
....
....
....
....
....
....
....
....
....
....
....
....
....
....
....
....
....

Shopping List ②

....
....
....
....
....
....
....
....
....
....
....
....
....
....
....
....
....
....
....

Four

CHANGE +/-   CURRENT WEIGHT

— *The Week Ahead* —

REMINDERS FOR THIS WEEK

LAST WEEK, THESE THINGS WENT WELL...

IN THE FREEZER   DATE   FOOD TO USE UP   DATE

MELTY BACON *and* CHEESE PORK BURGERS

Raw patties and melty toppers only

⏱ **20 MINS*** | 🍲 **15 MINS** | ✕ **SERVES 4**
*PLUS 15 MINS CHILLING

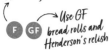

F GF → *Use GF bread rolls and Henderson's relish*

PER SERVING
449 KCAL / 31G CARBS

FOR THE MELTY TOPPERS
low-calorie cooking spray
4 smoked bacon
  medallions, diced
  (unsmoked works too)
125g low-fat spreadable
  cheese
40g reduced-fat Cheddar,
  finely grated
½ tsp sweet smoked
  paprika

FOR THE BURGER PATTIES
500g 5%-fat minced pork
½ tsp sweet smoked
  paprika
½ tsp garlic granules or
  powder
½ tsp English mustard
  powder
1 tbsp Henderson's relish or
  Worcestershire sauce
1 tbsp tomato puree
sea salt and freshly ground
  black pepper

Who doesn't love burger night? If you can't resist a bacon cheeseburger, this recipe is for you! We've switched beef patties for lean pork, and added some seriously cheesy, melty toppers to take your burger to the next level. You can even try sizzling them on the barbecue in the summer.

Special Occasion

Spray a frying pan with low-calorie cooking spray and place over a medium heat. Add the diced bacon medallions and cook for 5 minutes until cooked through. Set aside.

While the bacon is cooling, mix all the ingredients for the patties in a bowl and season with salt and pepper. It's best to mix everything with your hands as this helps to bring the meat together.

Shape the mixture into 4 patties and leave to rest in the fridge for 15 minutes.

While the burger patties are in the fridge, mix all the melty topper ingredients together in a bowl. The mixture should be very thick and sticky. Using clean hands, shape it into 4 small patty shapes and place in the fridge. (At this stage you could individually wrap and freeze the burger patties and the melty toppers for another day.)

Remove the burger patties from the fridge. Spray a frying pan with low-calorie cooking spray and place over a medium heat.

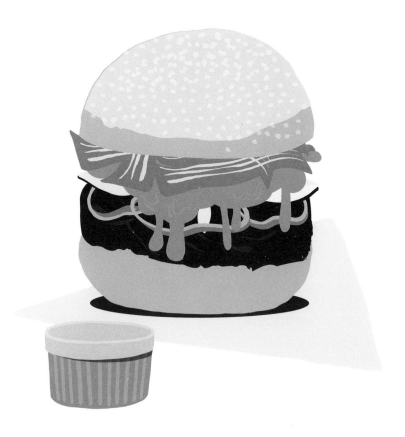

FOR THE BURGERS
4 wholemeal rolls (60g each), sliced in half
1 large tomato, thinly sliced
handful of salad leaves

TO ACCOMPANY *(optional)*
75g mixed salad (+ 15 kcal per serving)

When the pan is hot, add the burgers and fry for about 5 minutes on each side or until cooked through. If using a barbecue, spray the burgers with low-calorie cooking spray before placing them on the hot griddle to cook.

When the burgers are nearly done, pop a melty topper on top of each patty and let it melt. Now assemble your burgers: add a patty, some tomato slices and salad leaves to each roll and serve.

Weekly Meal Planner

	BREAKFAST	LUNCH
MONDAY		
TUESDAY		
WEDNESDAY		
THURSDAY		
FRIDAY		
SATURDAY		
SUNDAY		

Weekly Meal Planner

DINNER	SNACK	NOTES

Day One

BREAKFAST	VALUES
TOTAL	

LUNCH	VALUES
TOTAL	

DINNER	VALUES
TOTAL	

SNACKS AND TREATS	VALUES
TOTAL	
DAILY TOTAL	

WATER

Notes

Day Two

BREAKFAST	VALUES
TOTAL	

LUNCH	VALUES
TOTAL	

DINNER	VALUES
TOTAL	

SNACKS AND TREATS	VALUES
TOTAL	
DAILY TOTAL	

WATER

'It's all scribble and marks but that's what a planner is for, right? As someone much cleverer than me said "To fail to plan is to plan to fail" and so far, I'm not failing.' **ANGIE**

CURRIED FISH PIE

🕐 **15 MINS** | 🍲 **1 HOUR** | ✕ **SERVES 4**

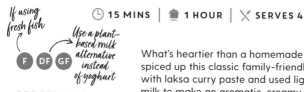

If using fresh fish

Use a plant-based milk alternative instead of yoghurt

(F) (DF) (GF)

PER SERVING
499 KCAL / 52G CARBS

SPECIAL EQUIPMENT
24 x 36cm (9½ x 14in)
ovenproof dish

FOR THE PIE TOPPING
800g floury potatoes
   such as Maris Piper or
   King Edward, peeled
   and cut into chunks
75g fat-free natural
   yoghurt
good handful of fresh
   coriander, roughly
   chopped

FOR THE PIE FILLING
low-calorie cooking spray
1 small onion, peeled and
   finely diced
1 x 185g jar laksa curry
   paste
1 x 400g tin light coconut
   milk
150g butternut squash,
   peeled, seeds removed
   and cut into 1cm (½in)
   dice (prepared weight)
100g fine green beans,
   trimmed and cut
   into thirds
400g mixed fish, cut into
   2cm (¾in) chunks
75g frozen peas
sea salt

What's heartier than a homemade fish pie? We've spiced up this classic family-friendly comfort dish with laksa curry paste and used light coconut milk to make an aromatic, creamy filling with a delicate spice that brings out all the flavours in the fish. Using shop-bought fish pie mix saves on time. Budget friendly, slimming friendly and so tasty!

Weekly Indulgence ─────────────

Place the potatoes in a pan of cold salted water and bring to the boil over a high heat. Reduce the heat and simmer for 20–25 minutes until soft.

Drain the potatoes and return to the pan. Mash until smooth, then mix in the yoghurt and coriander until thoroughly combined.

Preheat the oven to 190°C.

While the potatoes are cooking, prepare the pie filling. Spray a large, deep frying pan or wok with low-calorie cooking spray and place over a medium heat.

Add the onion and fry for 5 minutes until soft, then add the laksa paste and cook for 1 minute, stirring well. Pour in the coconut milk and 100ml water and add the butternut squash. Bring to the boil, then reduce the heat and simmer for 10 minutes.

Add the green beans and continue to simmer for a further 15 minutes, until the butternut squash is soft, the beans are cooked and the sauce has thickened slightly.

Stir in the fish and frozen peas and transfer the mix to the ovenproof dish. Spoon the mashed potato evenly on top, taking care to spread it right to the

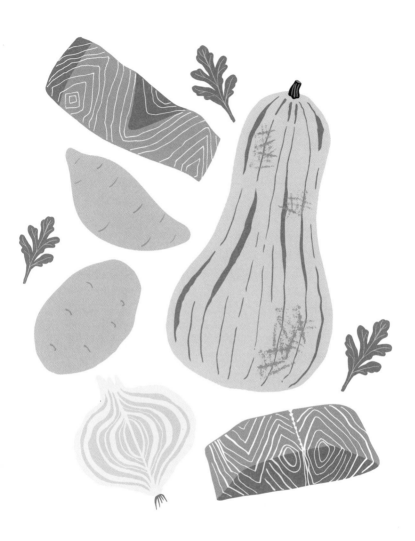

TO ACCOMPANY *(optional)*

80g steamed green
vegetables (+ 35 kcal
per serving)

edges to seal. Use a fork to add texture to the
surface of the mash.

Place in the oven and cook for 25 minutes until the
fish is opaque and thoroughly cooked through and
the top is golden. Serve with an accompaniment of
your choice.

Day Three

BREAKFAST	VALUES
TOTAL	

LUNCH	VALUES
TOTAL	

DINNER	VALUES
TOTAL	

SNACKS AND TREATS	VALUES
TOTAL	
DAILY TOTAL	

WATER

○ ○ ○ ○
○ ○ ○ ○

Notes

Day Four

BREAKFAST	VALUES
TOTAL	

LUNCH	VALUES
TOTAL	

DINNER	VALUES
TOTAL	

SNACKS AND TREATS	VALUES
TOTAL	
DAILY TOTAL	

WATER

○ ○ ○ ○
○ ○ ○ ○

Notes

Day Five

BREAKFAST	VALUES
TOTAL	

LUNCH	VALUES
TOTAL	

DINNER	VALUES
TOTAL	

SNACKS AND TREATS	VALUES
TOTAL	
DAILY TOTAL	

WATER

○ ○ ○ ○
○ ○ ○ ○

Notes

COOKING *WITH* LOVE PROVIDES FOOD *FOR THE* Soul

Day Six

BREAKFAST	VALUES
TOTAL	

LUNCH	VALUES
TOTAL	

DINNER	VALUES
TOTAL	

SNACKS AND TREATS	VALUES
TOTAL	
DAILY TOTAL	

WATER

Notes

Day Seven

BREAKFAST	VALUES
TOTAL	

LUNCH	VALUES
TOTAL	

DINNER	VALUES
TOTAL	

SNACKS AND TREATS	VALUES
TOTAL	
DAILY TOTAL	

WATER

◇ ◇ ◇ ◇
◇ ◇ ◇ ◇

Notes

CHANGE +/-   CURRENT WEIGHT

— *The Week Ahead* ————————————

REMINDERS FOR THIS WEEK

LAST WEEK, THESE THINGS WENT WELL...

IN THE FREEZER   DATE   FOOD TO USE UP   DATE

CREAMY PEPPERCORN MEATBALLS

Use GF breadcrumbs, stock pot and Henderson's relish

🕐 **15 MINS** | 🍲 **35 MINS** | ✕ **SERVES 4**

Use non-dairy cream cheese

PER SERVING
255 KCAL / 8.5G CARBS

FOR THE MEATBALLS
25g wholemeal bread
500g extra-lean minced beef
½ onion, peeled and very finely chopped
½ tsp garlic granules
½ tsp dried thyme
2 tsp Henderson's relish or Worcestershire sauce
1 medium egg, beaten
a good pinch of salt

FOR THE SAUCE
low-calorie cooking spray
½ onion, peeled and sliced
75g mushrooms, sliced
½ tsp cracked black pepper
500ml beef stock (1 beef stock pot dissolved in 500ml boiling water)
150g low-fat cream cheese

TO ACCOMPANY (optional)
80g steamed green vegetables (+ 35 kcal per serving)

Meatballs are a go-to teatime classic. The creamy, homemade peppercorn sauce gives these meatballs a satisfying peppery bite. We've kept the calories low using extra-lean mince and low-fat cream cheese. Serve them up with mashed potatoes and veggies for an instant winter warmer you can batch cook!

Everyday Light ————————————————

Use a food processor to blitz the bread into fine breadcrumbs. Place in a medium bowl with the rest of the meatball ingredients and mix well until thoroughly combined. Divide into twelve even pieces and roll into firm balls.

Spray a frying pan with low-calorie cooking spray and place over a medium-high heat. When the pan is hot, add the meatballs and fry for 2–3 minutes until brown on all sides (they don't need to be cooked through at this stage). You may find it easier to fry the meatballs in two batches if your pan is small. When nicely browned, remove from the pan and set to one side.

Now, make the sauce. Wipe out the pan and spray it again with low-calorie cooking spray. Reduce the heat to medium, add the onion and mushrooms and sauté for 5 minutes until beginning to soften. Stir in the cracked black pepper and cook for 1 minute. Add the stock then whisk in the cream cheese. Return the meatballs to the pan, bring to a simmer and cook for 10 minutes, then turn the meatballs over and simmer for a further 10 minutes.

Check the consistency of the sauce. If it is too runny, continue cooking for a few more minutes until it is the consistency of single cream and coats the meatballs. Serve with your choice of accompaniment.

75

Weekly Meal Planner

	BREAKFAST	LUNCH
MONDAY		
TUESDAY		
WEDNESDAY		
THURSDAY		
FRIDAY		
SATURDAY		
SUNDAY		

Weekly Meal Planner

DINNER	SNACK	NOTES

Day One

BREAKFAST	VALUES
TOTAL	

LUNCH	VALUES
TOTAL	

DINNER	VALUES
TOTAL	

SNACKS AND TREATS	VALUES
TOTAL	
DAILY TOTAL	

WATER

○ ○ ○ ○
○ ○ ○ ○

Notes

Day Two

BREAKFAST	VALUES
TOTAL	

LUNCH	VALUES
TOTAL	

DINNER	VALUES
TOTAL	

SNACKS AND TREATS	VALUES
TOTAL	
DAILY TOTAL	

WATER

○ ○ ○ ○
○ ○ ○ ○

Notes

Day Three

BREAKFAST	VALUES
TOTAL	

LUNCH	VALUES
TOTAL	

DINNER	VALUES
TOTAL	

SNACKS AND TREATS	VALUES
TOTAL	
DAILY TOTAL	

WATER

○ ○ ○ ○
○ ○ ○ ○

Notes

Day Four

BREAKFAST	VALUES
TOTAL	

LUNCH	VALUES
TOTAL	

DINNER	VALUES
TOTAL	

SNACKS AND TREATS	VALUES
TOTAL	
DAILY TOTAL	

WATER

○ ○ ○ ○
○ ○ ○ ○

Notes

PESTO PASTA BAKE

🕐 **25 MINS** | 🍲 **1 HOUR 20 MINS** | ✕ **SERVES 6**

Use GF pasta and sausages

F **BF** **GF**

PER SERVING
367 KCAL / 42G CARBS

SPECIAL EQUIPMENT
large (about 27cm /
10½in) ovenproof dish

24 large, dried pasta shells
  (about 240g)
6 low-fat pork sausages,
  quartered
70g reduced-fat
  mozzarella, cut into
  small chunks
30g Parmesan, finely
  grated
sea salt and freshly ground
  black pepper
a few fresh basil leaves,
  to garnish (optional)

FOR THE TOMATO SAUCE
low-calorie cooking spray
1 medium onion, peeled
  and finely diced
2 garlic cloves, peeled and
  crushed
1 x 400g tin chopped
  tomatoes
500g passata
2 tsp dried basil
1 tsp granulated sweetener
  or caster sugar

Everyone loves a cheese-topped pasta bake!
We've used low-fat meatballs and a homemade
green pesto sauce to fill these supersized shells.
They're oven baked until golden in a rich, tomato
sauce with a melty mozzarella and Parmesan
topping. You can even save a portion or two for
another day – this dish freezes really well.

Everyday Light ———————————

Cook the pasta shells in a large saucepan of
boiling water for 8–10 minutes, or according to the
packet instructions, until tender when a sharp knife
is inserted. Take care not to overcook them, as the
shells may become mushy. Drain well, then lay the
shells out on a chopping board so they don't stick
together. Set aside.

While the pasta shells are cooking, make the
tomato sauce. Spray a large frying pan with low-
calorie cooking spray and place over a medium
heat. Add the onion and fry for 5 minutes until
softened. Add the garlic and continue to fry for
a further 2 minutes. Add the chopped tomatoes,
passata, dried basil, sweetener or sugar and
season well with salt and pepper. Stir well, cover
and simmer gently over a medium-low heat for
20–25 minutes until the sauce has thickened
slightly. Pour the tomato sauce into the ovenproof
dish and spread out evenly. Set aside.

Now make the pesto sauce. Blend the basil
leaves, garlic, pine nuts, Parmesan, lemon juice
and 3 tablespoons of cold water together in a
food processor, or use a stick blender to blitz
them together in a bowl until it's a smooth, soft
consistency. Add a little more water if needed.
Season to taste with salt and pepper. Set aside.
Preheat the oven to 220°C (fan 200°C/gas mark 7).

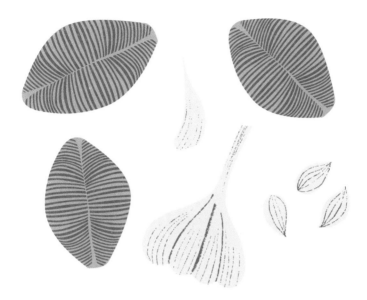

FOR THE PESTO SAUCE
50g fresh basil leaves
3 garlic cloves, peeled and
   crushed
35g pine nuts
15g Parmesan, finely grated
juice of ½ lemon

TO ACCOMPANY *(optional)*
75g mixed salad (+ 15 kcal
   per serving)

To make the sausage meatballs, wipe out the frying pan and spray it with low-calorie cooking spray. Place over a medium heat. Add the quartered sausages and fry gently for 13–15 minutes until cooked through and lightly browned.

To assemble the bake, take the cooked, cooled pasta shells and roughly spread the pesto sauce around the inside of each one using the back of a teaspoon. Place a cooked piece of sausage inside each pasta shell. Place the stuffed pasta shells in a single layer on top of the tomato sauce in the ovenproof dish. Scatter the mozzarella and Parmesan over the top. Place on a large baking tray and cover tightly with foil. Place in the oven for about 30 minutes or until piping hot throughout and golden. Remove the foil for the last 5 minutes to brown the top.

SWAP THIS:
Swap the pork sausages
for veggie sausages
if you prefer.

Scatter with a few fresh basil leaves (optional) and serve at once with an accompaniment of your choice.

Day Five

BREAKFAST	VALUES
TOTAL	

LUNCH	VALUES
TOTAL	

DINNER	VALUES
TOTAL	

SNACKS AND TREATS	VALUES
TOTAL	
DAILY TOTAL	

WATER

○ ○ ○ ○
○ ○ ○ ○

> 'I have the new planner and love the recipes . . .
> all the other books helped me so much in
> losing my weight.' **CHELLE**

Day Six

BREAKFAST	VALUES
TOTAL	

LUNCH	VALUES
TOTAL	

DINNER	VALUES
TOTAL	

SNACKS AND TREATS	VALUES
TOTAL	
DAILY TOTAL	

WATER

Notes

Day Seven

BREAKFAST	VALUES
TOTAL	

LUNCH	VALUES
TOTAL	

DINNER	VALUES
TOTAL	

SNACKS AND TREATS	VALUES
TOTAL	
DAILY TOTAL	

WATER

○ ○ ○ ○
○ ○ ○ ○

Notes

Shopping List ❶

....
....
....
....
....
....
....
....
....
....
....
....
....
....
....
....
....
....
....

Shopping List ❷

....
....
....
....
....
....
....
....
....
....
....
....
....
....
....
....
....
....
....

Shopping List ①

....
....
....
....
....
....
....
....
....
....
....
....
....
....
....
....
....
....

Shopping List ②

....
....
....
....
....
....
....
....
....
....
....
....
....
....
....
....
....
....

WEEK
Six

CHANGE +/-   **CURRENT WEIGHT**

— *The Week Ahead* ——————————————

REMINDERS FOR THIS WEEK

LAST WEEK, THESE THINGS WENT WELL...

IN THE FREEZER   DATE   **FOOD TO USE UP**   DATE

TORTILLA-TOPPED PASTA BAKE

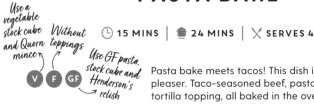

Use a vegetable stock cube and Quorn mince

Without toppings

Use GF pasta, stock cube and Henderson's relish

V F GF

🕐 **15 MINS** | 📦 **24 MINS** | ✕ **SERVES 4**

Pasta bake meets tacos! This dish is a total crowd-pleaser. Taco-seasoned beef, pasta and a cheesy tortilla topping, all baked in the oven and on the table in under 40 minutes. It's quick, easy and always a winner. You can add your own toppings or even leave out the tortilla chips altogether if you fancy a simple pasta dish.

PER SERVING
566 KCAL / 71G CARBS

SPECIAL EQUIPMENT
18 x 27cm (7 x 10½in) ovenproof dish

FOR THE TACO SEASONING
¼ tsp chilli powder
¼ tsp dried oregano
¼ tsp onion granules
¼ tsp garlic granules
¼ tsp smoked paprika
¼ tsp ground cumin

FOR THE MEAT SAUCE
low-calorie cooking spray
1 large onion, peeled and diced
3 garlic cloves, peeled and minced
250g 5%-fat minced beef
1 beef stock cube, crumbled
2 tbsp Henderson's relish or Worcestershire sauce
1½ tsp taco seasoning (above)
1 x 400g tin chopped tomatoes
1 x 400g tin mixed beans in tomato sauce
250g dried pasta shells or other pasta shapes
sea salt and freshly ground black pepper

Special Occasion

First, combine the taco seasoning ingredients in a bowl.

To make the meat sauce for the pasta, spray a frying pan with low-calorie cooking spray and place over a medium heat. Add the onion and garlic and cook gently for 5 minutes until they begin to soften.

Add the minced beef, crumbled stock cube and Henderson's relish to the pan and stir. Cook for another 5 minutes, breaking up the mince with a wooden spoon, until the beef is browned.

Add the taco seasoning, chopped tomatoes and beans, season with salt and pepper and stir well. Reduce the heat a little and simmer while you cook the pasta.

Preheat the oven to 220°C (fan 200°C/gas mark 7).

Cook the pasta according to the packet instructions (about 10–12 minutes).

When the pasta is cooked, drain it well and mix it with the meat sauce. Spoon the mixture evenly among four individual roasting dishes. We like to do this so everyone in the family can customise

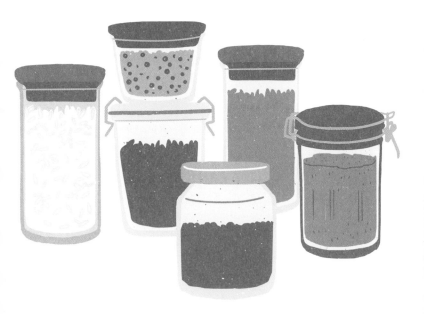

FOR THE TOPPINGS
40g reduced-fat Cheddar, finely grated
30g lightly salted tortilla chips, very finely crushed
70g sliced jalapeños in brine, drained, to serve

FOR THE CHEESE SAUCE
125g low-fat spreadable cheese
¼ tsp smoked paprika

TIP: If you want to opt for different toppings, the calories for the pasta and beef sauce without any cheese or toppings is 441 kcal per serving.

their toppings, but it will work fine as one large pasta bake too!

Sprinkle the cheese and tortilla chip crumbs evenly over the top and bake in the oven for 10 minutes until the cheese is melted and golden.

While the cheese is melting, mix the cheese sauce ingredients together with 3 tablespoons of water until smooth. If it seems too thick add a small splash of water at a time until you reach your preferred consistency.

When the bake is ready, drizzle over the cheese sauce, top with the sliced jalapeños and serve!

Weekly Meal Planner

	BREAKFAST	LUNCH
MONDAY		
TUESDAY		
WEDNESDAY		
THURSDAY		
FRIDAY		
SATURDAY		
SUNDAY		

Weekly Meal Planner

DINNER	SNACK	NOTES

Day One

BREAKFAST	VALUES
TOTAL	

LUNCH	VALUES
TOTAL	

DINNER	VALUES
TOTAL	

SNACKS AND TREATS	VALUES
TOTAL	
DAILY TOTAL	

WATER

Notes

CREAMY TUSCAN-STYLE SALMON

🕐 **10 MINS** | 🍲 **20 MINS** | ✕ **SERVES 4**

Use GF stock cube

GF

PER SERVING
500 KCAL / 9.6G CARBS

low-calorie cooking spray
300g cherry tomatoes,
   halved
1 medium onion, peeled
   and diced
3 garlic cloves, peeled and
   crushed
4 skinless, boneless salmon
   fillets (about 125g each)
200g low-fat cream
   cheese
150ml vegetable stock
   (1 vegetable stock cube
   dissolved in 150ml boiling
   water)
150ml low-fat double
   cream alternative
80g baby spinach, roughly
   chopped
sea salt and freshly ground
   black pepper

TO ACCOMPANY *(optional)*
80g steamed green
   vegetables (+ 35 kcal
   per serving)

Inspired by the flavours of Tuscany, this creamy salmon dish is lighter than you'd think. We've used roasted cherry tomatoes to add little bursts of sweetness to the rich, savoury sauce. Although it tastes luxurious, we've kept the calories low by using low-fat cream cheese and a low-fat double cream alternative. It's guaranteed to be a new family favourite!

Weekly Indulgence

Preheat the oven to 220°C (fan 200°C/gas mark 7). Spray a baking tray with low-calorie cooking spray, add the cherry tomatoes and arrange them cut side up in a single layer, and roast in the oven for 15 minutes until the skin is wrinkled.

While the tomatoes are in the oven, spray a large frying pan with low-calorie cooking spray and place over a medium heat. Add the onion and fry for 4 minutes until just softening, then add the garlic and fry for a further 2 minutes.

While the onion is cooking, spray another frying pan with low-calorie cooking spray and place over a medium heat. Add the salmon and fry for 3 minutes on each side, then set aside.

Add the cream cheese and stock to the pan of onion and garlic and stir until the cream cheese is fully incorporated. Stir in the double cream alternative and add the spinach.

Once the tomatoes are cooked, remove from the oven and add to the pan. Reduce the heat to a simmer, add the salmon fillets and simmer for a few minutes until they are cooked through. Season with salt and pepper and serve with your choice of accompaniment.

Day Two

BREAKFAST	VALUES
TOTAL	

LUNCH	VALUES
TOTAL	

DINNER	VALUES
TOTAL	

SNACKS AND TREATS	VALUES
TOTAL	
DAILY TOTAL	

WATER

⬡ ⬡ ⬡ ⬡
⬡ ⬡ ⬡ ⬡

Notes

Day Three

BREAKFAST	VALUES
TOTAL	

LUNCH	VALUES
TOTAL	

DINNER	VALUES
TOTAL	

SNACKS AND TREATS	VALUES
TOTAL	
DAILY TOTAL	

WATER

○ ○ ○ ○
○ ○ ○ ○

'I treated myself to a Pinch of Nom recipe book and food planner diary. I'll be meal planning AND PREPPING because it's the prepping that works for me!' **GINA**

Day Four

BREAKFAST	VALUES
TOTAL	

LUNCH	VALUES
TOTAL	

DINNER	VALUES
TOTAL	

SNACKS AND TREATS	VALUES
TOTAL	
DAILY TOTAL	

WATER

○ ○ ○ ○
○ ○ ○ ○

Notes

Day Five

BREAKFAST	VALUES
TOTAL	

LUNCH	VALUES
TOTAL	

DINNER	VALUES
TOTAL	

SNACKS AND TREATS	VALUES
TOTAL	
DAILY TOTAL	

WATER

△△△△
△△△△

Notes

Day Six

BREAKFAST	VALUES
TOTAL	

LUNCH	VALUES
TOTAL	

DINNER	VALUES
TOTAL	

SNACKS AND TREATS	VALUES
TOTAL	
DAILY TOTAL	

WATER

Notes

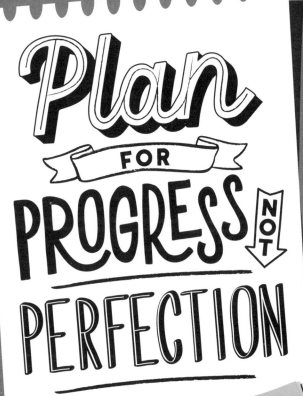

Day Seven

BREAKFAST	VALUES
TOTAL	

LUNCH	VALUES
TOTAL	

DINNER	VALUES
TOTAL	

SNACKS AND TREATS	VALUES
TOTAL	
DAILY TOTAL	

WATER

Notes

HIDDEN VEG FRITTERS

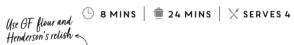

⏱ **8 MINS** | 🍲 **24 MINS** | ✕ **SERVES 4**

Use GF flour and Henderson's relish ←

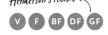

PER SERVING (2 FRITTERS)
138 KCAL / 19G CARBS

120g butternut squash, peeled, deseeded and cut into 2cm (¾in) cubes
low-calorie cooking spray
½ medium onion, peeled and diced
1 x 400g tin butter beans, drained and rinsed
60g sweetcorn (tinned or frozen and cooked)
60g frozen peas
¼ tsp garlic granules
¼ tsp onion granules
½ tsp smoked paprika
1 tsp tomato puree
¼ tsp Henderson's relish or Worcestershire sauce
1 medium egg, beaten
20g plain flour
sea salt and freshly ground black pepper

These fritters are a slimming-friendly way to use up leftover veg. They're great as a snack or as an addition to a main meal, quick to prep and help towards your five a day. The beauty of this recipe is that it works with an endless combination of veggies – here we've thrown together a tasty blend of butternut squash, peas, sweetcorn and onion.

Everyday Light

Put the butternut squash in a microwavable bowl and cover loosely with cling film. Cook for 3 minutes until the squash is soft. Alternatively, cook the squash in a pan of water over a medium heat for about 10–12 minutes until soft. Leave to one side to cool slightly.

Spray a frying pan with low-calorie cooking spray and place over a medium-low heat. Add the onion and sauté for 3 minutes until lightly golden and softened.

Put the butter beans, sweetcorn, peas, cooked butternut squash and onion in a food processor and blitz until coarsely chopped. Tip the vegetables into the bowl and add the garlic granules, onion granules, paprika, tomato puree and Henderson's relish. Season with salt and pepper, add the egg and flour, and mix until fully combined.

Spray a frying pan with low-calorie cooking spray and place over a medium heat. Add 2–3 tablespoons of the fritter mixture to the pan and flatten out slightly: depending on the size of your pan you can cook two or three fritters at a time. Cook for 3 minutes on each side until golden brown. Repeat with the rest of the fritter mixture – the mixture should make eight fritters in total.

Seven

CHANGE +/-   **CURRENT WEIGHT**

— The Week Ahead —

REMINDERS FOR THIS WEEK

LAST WEEK, THESE THINGS WENT WELL...

IN THE FREEZER   DATE   **FOOD TO USE UP**   DATE

CREAMY BALSAMIC CHICKEN *and* MUSHROOMS

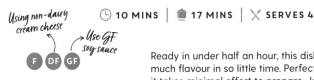

🕐 **10 MINS** | 🍲 **17 MINS** | ✕ **SERVES 4**

Using non-dairy cream cheese

Use GF soy sauce

F **DF** **GF**

PER SERVING
192 KCAL / 16G CARBS

300g button mushrooms, quartered

2 garlic cloves, peeled and crushed

400g skinless chicken breasts (about 2 breasts), cut into 3cm (1¼in)-wide strips

3 tbsp balsamic vinegar

2 tbsp dark soy sauce

2 tbsp honey

4 tbsp low-fat cream cheese

4g fresh parsley, chopped

Ready in under half an hour, this dish builds up so much flavour in so little time. Perfect for busy days, it takes minimal effort to prepare. Just pop all the ingredients into a pan and leave them to bubble away while you make mashed potatoes, cook fresh vegetables or prepare a crisp side salad to serve it with. Simple and delicious!

Everyday Light ———————————————

Set a large frying pan over a medium-low heat, add the mushrooms and fry for 4 minutes until they have softened and the moisture they release has begun to reduce. Add the garlic and chicken and cook for about 5 minutes, to brown the chicken on all sides.

Add the balsamic vinegar, soy sauce and honey and reduce the heat to a simmer.

Allow the mixture to bubble gently for 8 minutes, until the sauce has reduced and the chicken is thoroughly cooked through and shows no sign of pinkness.

Remove from the heat and stir through the cream cheese until the chicken and mushrooms are coated and the cream cheese has melted and become smooth. Stir through the chopped parsley and serve.

Weekly Meal Planner

	BREAKFAST	LUNCH
MONDAY		
TUESDAY		
WEDNESDAY		
THURSDAY		
FRIDAY		
SATURDAY		
SUNDAY		

Weekly Meal Planner

DINNER	SNACK	NOTES

Day One

BREAKFAST	VALUES
TOTAL	

LUNCH	VALUES
TOTAL	

DINNER	VALUES
TOTAL	

SNACKS AND TREATS	VALUES
TOTAL	
DAILY TOTAL	

WATER

○ ○ ○ ○
○ ○ ○ ○

Notes

Day Two

BREAKFAST	VALUES
TOTAL	

LUNCH	VALUES
TOTAL	

DINNER	VALUES
TOTAL	

SNACKS AND TREATS	VALUES
TOTAL	
DAILY TOTAL	

WATER

◊ ◊ ◊ ◊
◊ ◊ ◊ ◊

Notes

Day Three

BREAKFAST	VALUES
TOTAL	

LUNCH	VALUES
TOTAL	

DINNER	VALUES
TOTAL	

SNACKS AND TREATS	VALUES
TOTAL	
DAILY TOTAL	

WATER

◊ ◊ ◊ ◊
◊ ◊ ◊ ◊

Notes

Day Four

BREAKFAST	VALUES
TOTAL	

LUNCH	VALUES
TOTAL	

DINNER	VALUES
TOTAL	

SNACKS AND TREATS	VALUES
TOTAL	
DAILY TOTAL	

WATER

○ ○ ○ ○
○ ○ ○ ○

Notes

Day Five

BREAKFAST	VALUES
TOTAL	

LUNCH	VALUES
TOTAL	

DINNER	VALUES
TOTAL	

SNACKS AND TREATS	VALUES
TOTAL	
DAILY TOTAL	

WATER

'Absolutely love my planner, thank you!'
SAMANTHA

Day Six

BREAKFAST	VALUES
TOTAL	

LUNCH	VALUES
TOTAL	

DINNER	VALUES
TOTAL	

SNACKS AND TREATS	VALUES
TOTAL	
DAILY TOTAL	

WATER

Notes

CAULIFLOWER CHEESE SOUP

Use a GF / veggie stock cube and Henderson's relish

without bacon

V F BF GF

🕐 10 MINS | 🍲 40 MINS | ✗ SERVES 6

PER SERVING
210 KCAL / 18G CARBS

low-calorie cooking spray
1 medium onion, peeled
    and diced
2 garlic cloves, peeled and
    crushed
1 medium carrot, peeled
    and sliced
1 celery stick, diced
500g cauliflower, leaves
    discarded and florets
    broken into small pieces
1 medium potato, peeled
    and diced
600ml chicken or
    vegetable stock
    (1 chicken or vegetable
    stock cube dissolved in
    600ml boiling water)
2 bacon medallions, cut
    into thin strips
2 tsp Dijon mustard
¼ tsp chilli powder
1 tsp sriracha sauce
1 tsp Worcestershire sauce
    or Henderson's relish
130g reduced-fat mature
    Cheddar, grated
4 tbsp low-fat cream
    cheese
sea salt and freshly ground
    black pepper
a few chives, chopped,
    to garnish

This twist on classic cauliflower cheese might just be our new favourite soup for chilly evenings. We've packed plenty of secret veggies into this hearty soup, so it's extra filling, and it'll help you on your way to your five-a-day too. You won't believe there's no cream in the recipe – it's so cheesy and tastes indulgent, while still being low in calories.

Everyday Light ———————————

Spray a large saucepan with low-calorie cooking spray and place over a medium heat. Add the onion and fry for 4 minutes until starting to soften, then add the garlic, carrot and celery and fry for xa further 2 minutes.

Add the cauliflower florets and potato to the saucepan along with the stock. Cover with a lid and simmer for 30 minutes until the vegetables are soft and cooked through.

While the vegetables are cooking, spray a small frying pan with low-calorie cooking spray and fry the bacon over a medium heat for a couple of minutes until crisp. Remove from the heat and leave to one side.

Once the vegetables are cooked, add the Dijon mustard, chilli powder, sriracha sauce and Worcestershire sauce or Henderson's relish, and give the mixture a good stir.

Using a stick blender in the pan, or a food processor, blitz the soup until smooth. You may need to do this in batches.

Add the grated Cheddar and cream cheese to the soup and stir until fully incorporated. If the soup is a

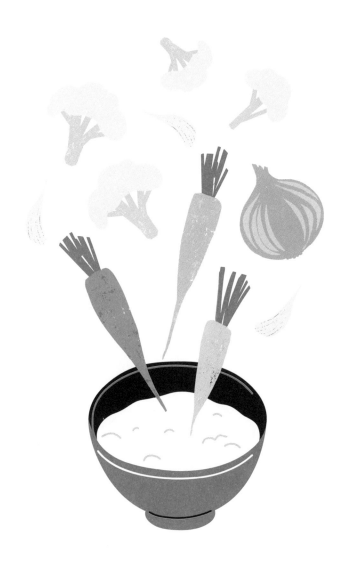

TO ACCOMPANY *(optional)*
60g wholemeal bread rolls
(+ 152 kcal per roll)

little thick, add a splash of boiling water. Season to taste with salt and pepper.

Serve in warm bowls sprinkled with the chives and crispy bacon.

Day Seven

BREAKFAST	VALUES
TOTAL	

LUNCH	VALUES
TOTAL	

DINNER	VALUES
TOTAL	

SNACKS AND TREATS	VALUES
TOTAL	
DAILY TOTAL	

WATER

○ ○ ○ ○
○ ○ ○ ○

Notes

Shopping List 1

....
....
....
....
....
....
....
....
....
....
....
....
....
....
....
....
....
....
....
....

Shopping List 2

....
....
....
....
....
....
....
....
....
....
....
....
....
....
....
....
....
....
....
....

Shopping List 1

....
....
....
....
....
....
....
....
....
....
....
....
....
....
....
....
....
....

Shopping List 2

....
....
....
....
....
....
....
....
....
....
....
....
....
....
....
....
....
....

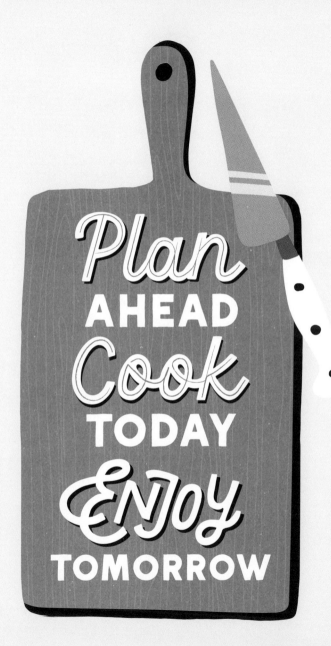

Eight

CHANGE +/- **CURRENT WEIGHT**

— The Week Ahead —

REMINDERS FOR THIS WEEK

LAST WEEK, THESE THINGS WENT WELL...

IN THE FREEZER DATE **FOOD TO USE UP** DATE

CHERRY BAKEWELL CRUMBLE

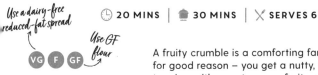

Use a dairy-free reduced-fat spread

Use GF flour

(VG) (F) (GF)

🕐 **20 MINS** | 🍲 **30 MINS** | ✗ **SERVES 6**

PER SERVING
301 KCAL* / 30G CARBS
*When using granulated
sweetener

SPECIAL EQUIPMENT
18 x 27cm ovenproof dish

400g frozen dark, sweet
    cherries
3 tbsp granulated sweetener
    or caster sugar
100g self-raising flour
50g reduced-fat spread
100g ground almonds
20g flaked almonds

TO ACCOMPANY *(optional)*
Custard (+ 58 kcal per
    serving)

A fruity crumble is a comforting family classic
for good reason – you get a nutty, golden
topping with sweet, syrupy fruit underneath. This
slimming-friendly pudding combines the flavours
of a cherry Bakewell and a classic crumble to
create a sweet treat that captures the best of
both desserts. We love it served with a good glug
of homemade custard!

Weekly Indulgence ───────────────

Preheat the oven to 210°C (fan 190°C/gas mark 6).

Put the frozen cherries in the ovenproof dish,
sprinkle over 1 tablespoon of the sweetener and stir
to coat. Leave to one side.

To make the crumble mixture, put the flour and
reduced-fat spread in a mixing bowl and rub the
mixture between your fingers until it resembles
breadcrumbs. Stir in the remaining 2 tablespoons of
sweetener and the ground almonds.

Top the cherries with the crumble mixture and bake
in the oven for 15 minutes.

After 15 minutes, sprinkle the flaked almonds over
the crumble and cook for a further 15 minutes until
the crumble is lightly golden. Serve.

> **TIP:** To make custard, pour 375ml skimmed milk into a
> large saucepan. Heat over a medium heat until it just starts
> to steam. Do not let it burn the bottom of the pan or come
> to the boil. Mix 2 egg yolks, 1 tbsp cornflour and 3 tbsp
> granulated sweetener in a heatproof jug to form a smooth
> paste. Pour the hot milk into the jug and quickly stir it all
> together. Pour the mixture back into the pan and cook very
> slowly, stirring continuously, for 5–10 minutes until thick and
> starting to bubble. Leave to stand for 1 minute before serving.

Weekly Meal Planner

	BREAKFAST	LUNCH
MONDAY		
TUESDAY		
WEDNESDAY		
THURSDAY		
FRIDAY		
SATURDAY		
SUNDAY		

Weekly Meal Planner

DINNER	SNACK	NOTES

Day One

BREAKFAST	VALUES
TOTAL	

LUNCH	VALUES
TOTAL	

DINNER	VALUES
TOTAL	

SNACKS AND TREATS	VALUES
TOTAL	
DAILY TOTAL	

WATER

○ ○ ○ ○
○ ○ ○ ○

Notes

Day Two

BREAKFAST	VALUES
TOTAL	

LUNCH	VALUES
TOTAL	

DINNER	VALUES
TOTAL	

SNACKS AND TREATS	VALUES
TOTAL	
DAILY TOTAL	

WATER

○ ○ ○ ○
○ ○ ○ ○

Notes

Be proud
of every
small step
towards your
big goal

Day Three

BREAKFAST	VALUES
TOTAL	

LUNCH	VALUES
TOTAL	

DINNER	VALUES
TOTAL	

SNACKS AND TREATS	VALUES
TOTAL	
DAILY TOTAL	

WATER

Notes

Day Four

BREAKFAST	VALUES
TOTAL	

LUNCH	VALUES
TOTAL	

DINNER	VALUES
TOTAL	

SNACKS AND TREATS	VALUES
TOTAL	
DAILY TOTAL	

WATER

○ ○ ○ ○
○ ○ ○ ○

Notes

Day Five

BREAKFAST	VALUES
TOTAL	

LUNCH	VALUES
TOTAL	

DINNER	VALUES
TOTAL	

SNACKS AND TREATS	VALUES
TOTAL	
DAILY TOTAL	

WATER

◇ ◇ ◇ ◇
◇ ◇ ◇ ◇

'Nothing like buying a Pinch of Nom planner just for the extra recipes!' **KIRSTY**

RED VELVET WAFFLES

Use dairy-free yoghurt, cream cheese and aerosol cream

🕐 **5 MINS** | 🍲 **18 MINS** | ✕ **SERVES 2**

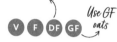 *Use GF oats*

PER SERVING
468 KCAL* / 58G CARBS
*When using granulated sweetener

SPECIAL EQUIPMENT
waffle maker

80g rolled oats
2 tbsp cocoa powder
1 tbsp white granulated
  sweetener or caster
  sugar
1 medium egg, beaten
350g fat-free natural
  yoghurt
1 tsp red food colouring
low-calorie cooking spray
40g low-fat cream cheese
1 tsp icing sugar

TO SERVE
20g milk chocolate chips
low-fat aerosol cream

How do you like your waffles in the morning? We like ours fluffy and light, with a touch of sweetness! This recipe has all the signature creamy red velvet flavours without the calories. Enjoy them fresh out of the oven as a sweet snack, brunch or breakfast. They are perfect finished with a drizzle of cream cheese and a swirl of aerosol cream.

Special Occasion

Preheat your waffle maker.

Blitz the oats to a fine consistency in a food processor.

Transfer the oats to a large mixing bowl and add the cocoa powder, sweetener, egg, natural yoghurt and food colouring. Mix until everything is fully combined and you have a smooth batter.

Once your waffle maker is hot, spray it with a little low-calorie cooking spray. Pour some of the waffle batter onto the hot plate and spread it out. We made 6 waffles with the quantity of batter this recipe makes, but how many you make will depend on the size of your waffle maker.

Seal your waffle maker and cook for 5–6 minutes or until the waffle is crispy and golden brown around the edges. Place the waffles on a plate and cover with foil to keep warm while you cook the rest of the batter.

While the waffles are cooking, mix the cream cheese and icing sugar in a small bowl with 1 teaspoon of cold water until smooth.

Stack up the waffles on two serving plates and drizzle with the sweetened cream cheese mixture. Top with the chocolate chips and a swirl of aerosol cream. Serve!

Day Six

BREAKFAST	VALUES
TOTAL	

LUNCH	VALUES
TOTAL	

DINNER	VALUES
TOTAL	

SNACKS AND TREATS	VALUES
TOTAL	
DAILY TOTAL	

WATER

○ ○ ○ ○
○ ○ ○ ○

Notes

Day Seven

BREAKFAST	VALUES
TOTAL	

LUNCH	VALUES
TOTAL	

DINNER	VALUES
TOTAL	

SNACKS AND TREATS	VALUES
TOTAL	
DAILY TOTAL	

WATER

Notes

Nine

CHANGE +/-   **CURRENT WEIGHT**

— The Week Ahead —

REMINDERS FOR THIS WEEK

LAST WEEK, THESE THINGS WENT WELL...

IN THE FREEZER   DATE   **FOOD TO USE UP**   DATE

VEGETABLE KORMA

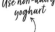

🕐 **15 MINS** | 🍲 **40 MINS** | ✕ **SERVES 4**

Use non-dairy yoghurt

PER SERVING
270 KCAL / 39G CARBS

low-calorie cooking spray
1 medium onion, peeled
   and chopped
2 garlic cloves, peeled and
   crushed
2cm (¾in) piece of root
   ginger, peeled and grated
2 sweet potatoes, about
   400g in total, peeled and
   cut into 2cm (¾in) cubes
2 tbsp tomato puree
400ml coconut dairy-free
   milk alternative
2 tbsp ground almonds
250g cauliflower, leaves
   removed and cut into
   small florets (prepared
   weight)
125g broccoli, cut into small
   florets
100g fine green beans,
   trimmed and halved
200g fat-free natural yoghurt
sea salt, to taste

**FOR THE KORMA
SPICE MIX**

1 tsp ground coriander
1 tsp unsmoked paprika
1 tsp ground turmeric
½ tsp ground cumin
¼ tsp ground cardamom
¼ tsp ground cinnamon
¼ tsp ground black pepper
pinch of ground cloves
pinch of dried chilli flakes

Our veggie twist on this classic Indian-style recipe replaces the meat with extra vegetables, simmering them in a mild, delicately spiced korma curry sauce. Low in calories without compromising on flavour, it's a great choice for Fakeaway night with the family. You can easily make this recipe vegan too – just switch to a non-dairy yoghurt.

Everyday Light

Combine the korma spice ingredients in a small bowl.

Spray a large frying pan with low-calorie cooking spray and place over a medium heat.

Add the onion and fry for 5 minutes until softening and golden, then add the garlic, ginger, and prepared korma spice mix. Cook for 1–2 minutes, stirring well. Stir in the sweet potato, tomato puree and coconut dairy-free milk alternative, reduce the heat, cover and simmer gently for 20 minutes, until the sweet potato is just tender.

Stir in the ground almonds and cauliflower florets, cover and simmer for 10 minutes, until the cauliflower is just tender (take care not to overcook it), then add the broccoli and beans, cover and cook for 3–4 minutes until all the vegetables are tender but not overcooked.

Stir in the yoghurt until evenly blended. Taste and season with salt if needed. Serve with your choice of accompaniment.

FOOD

is the

INGREDIENT

that brings us

together

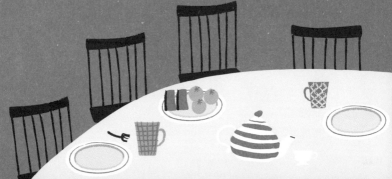

Weekly Meal Planner

	BREAKFAST	LUNCH
MONDAY		
TUESDAY		
WEDNESDAY		
THURSDAY		
FRIDAY		
SATURDAY		
SUNDAY		

Weekly Meal Planner

DINNER	SNACK	NOTES

Day One

BREAKFAST	VALUES
TOTAL	

LUNCH	VALUES
TOTAL	

DINNER	VALUES
TOTAL	

SNACKS AND TREATS	VALUES
TOTAL	
DAILY TOTAL	

WATER

○ ○ ○ ○
○ ○ ○ ○

Notes

Day Two

BREAKFAST	VALUES
TOTAL	

LUNCH	VALUES
TOTAL	

DINNER	VALUES
TOTAL	

SNACKS AND TREATS	VALUES
TOTAL	
DAILY TOTAL	

WATER

○ ○ ○ ○
○ ○ ○ ○

Notes

Day Three

BREAKFAST	VALUES
TOTAL	

LUNCH	VALUES
TOTAL	

DINNER	VALUES
TOTAL	

SNACKS AND TREATS	VALUES
TOTAL	
DAILY TOTAL	

WATER

◇ ◇ ◇ ◇
◇ ◇ ◇ ◇

Notes

Day Four

BREAKFAST	VALUES
TOTAL	

LUNCH	VALUES
TOTAL	

DINNER	VALUES
TOTAL	

SNACKS AND TREATS	VALUES
TOTAL	
DAILY TOTAL	

WATER

○ ○ ○ ○
○ ○ ○ ○

Notes

APPLE CINNAMON SWIRL PUDDING

Use vegan pastry and non-dairy milk

🕐 **20 MINS** | 🍲 **50 MINS** | ✕ **SERVES 6**

VG F

PER SERVING
270 KCAL* / 42G CARBS
*When using granulated sweetener

SPECIAL EQUIPMENT
18 x 27cm (7 x 10½in) ovenproof dish

4 tbsp granulated sweetener or caster sugar
¼ tsp ground cinnamon
600g cooking apples, peeled, cored and thinly sliced

FOR THE PASTRY TOP
320g ready-rolled light puff pastry sheet
2 tbsp granulated sweetener or caster sugar
2 tsp ground cinnamon
1 tsp skimmed milk, for brushing

TO ACCOMPANY *(optional)*
Custard (+ 58 kcal per serving, see page 121 for recipe)

With simple flavours and an even simpler method, this apple pudding is an easy family favourite. We've swapped out the more traditional crumble or pastry lid topping for a warming crispy cinnamon-swirl crust. The light puff pastry keeps the calories down and gives our sweet, fruity filling a crunchy finish. Pour custard on top for added comfort!

Weekly Indulgence ────────────

Preheat the oven to 180°C (fan 160°C/gas mark 4).

Add the sweetener (or sugar) and cinnamon to a little bowl and stir to combine. Place the apple slices in the ovenproof dish, sprinkle over the sweetener and cinnamon mix and toss to coat. Add 2 tablespoons of cold water and cover the dish tightly with foil. Place on a baking tray and bake in the oven for about 30 minutes, or until the apples are just tender when a small, sharp knife is inserted. Remove the foil and stir halfway through, replacing the foil before you return the dish to the oven.

Remove the dish of apples from the oven, set aside, and increase the oven temperature to 200°C (fan 180°C/gas mark 5).

To prepare the pastry top, unroll the pastry sheet on a work surface, leaving it on the greaseproof paper packing. Brush the pastry sheet all over with a little cold water to moisten it, then sprinkle over the sweetener (or sugar) and cinnamon in an even layer, leaving a 1cm (½in) gap along one long edge. Roll the pastry up tightly starting from the long edge without the gap and using the greaseproof paper packing to help you. Keep rolling until you've made a 'Swiss roll'. When you've finished rolling the pastry up, make sure it's seam side down.

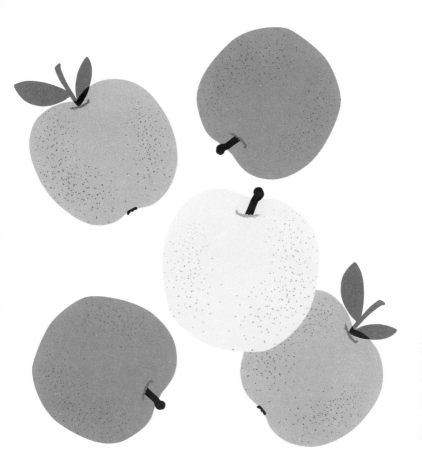

Use a large serrated knife to carefully cut it into 24 x 1cm (9½ x ½in)-wide spiral-shaped slices. Press the seam on each to ensure a good seal.

Remove the foil from the ovenproof dish and place the cinnamon swirls on top of the apples. It's fine to have small gaps between the cinnamon swirls as they will expand a little while baking. Brush the tops of the cinnamon swirls with the skimmed milk. Place the dish on the baking tray and bake in the oven for 20 minutes until the cinnamon swirls are golden and crispy, and the apples are soft. Serve hot with custard or another accompaniment.

TIP: Add a few raisins or sultanas to the apple filling if you like, and adjust the calories accordingly.

Day Five

BREAKFAST	VALUES
TOTAL	

LUNCH	VALUES
TOTAL	

DINNER	VALUES
TOTAL	

SNACKS AND TREATS	VALUES
TOTAL	
DAILY TOTAL	

WATER

'My planner has been a real help for keeping me on track and focused.' **CLAIRE**

Day Six

BREAKFAST	VALUES
TOTAL	

LUNCH	VALUES
TOTAL	

DINNER	VALUES
TOTAL	

SNACKS AND TREATS	VALUES
TOTAL	
DAILY TOTAL	

WATER

○ ○ ○ ○
○ ○ ○ ○

Notes

Day Seven

BREAKFAST	VALUES
TOTAL	

LUNCH	VALUES
TOTAL	

DINNER	VALUES
TOTAL	

SNACKS AND TREATS	VALUES
TOTAL	
DAILY TOTAL	

WATER

○ ○ ○ ○
○ ○ ○ ○

Notes

Shopping List 1

....
....
....
....
....
....
....
....
....
....
....
....
....
....
....
....
....
....
....

Shopping List 2

....
....
....
....
....
....
....
....
....
....
....
....
....
....
....
....
....
....

Shopping List ①

....
....
....
....
....
....
....
....
....
....
....
....
....
....
....
....
....
....

Shopping List ②

....
....
....
....
....
....
....
....
....
....
....
....
....
....
....
....
....
....

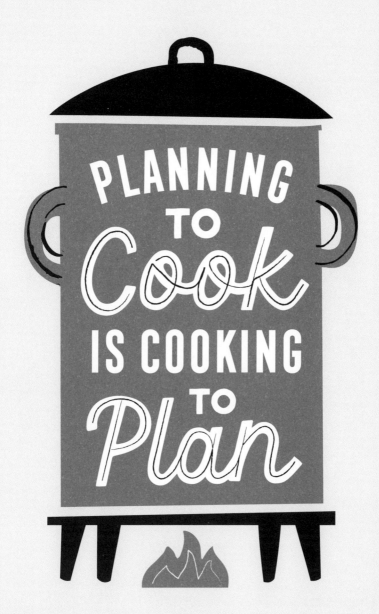

Ten

CHANGE +/- CURRENT WEIGHT

— The Week Ahead —

REMINDERS FOR THIS WEEK

LAST WEEK, THESE THINGS WENT WELL...

IN THE FREEZER DATE FOOD TO USE UP DATE

SAUSAGE *and* BAKED BEAN CHILLI

Use GF stock cubes, Henderson's relish and sausages ←

PER SERVING
228 KCAL / 25G CARBS

low-calorie cooking spray
1 large onion, peeled and
    diced
2 mixed peppers, deseeded
    and diced
2 carrots, peeled and diced
1 x 400g pack low-fat
    sausages, meat squeezed
    out of skins and skins
    discarded
3 garlic cloves, peeled and
    crushed
1 tbsp mild chilli powder
1 tsp smoked paprika
1 x 400g tin chopped
    tomatoes
400ml chicken stock
    (1 chicken stock cube
    dissolved in 400 ml
    boiling water)
1 tbsp tomato puree
1 tbsp Henderson's relish or
    Worcestershire sauce
1 x 420g tin baked beans

TO ACCOMPANY *(optional)*
50g raw basmati rice per
    portion, cooked
    according to packet
    instructions (+ 173 kcal per
    125g cooked serving)

Here's a midweek family dinner that'll warm you right up. Our Sausage and Baked Bean Chilli is a hearty mixture of fresh veggies and convenient store-cupboard ingredients. It's quick to prepare, easy to cook and super budget-friendly. Like with most batch-friendly chilli dishes, we guarantee the flavours will be even better the next day!

Everyday Light

Spray a large saucepan or deep frying pan with low-calorie cooking spray and place over a medium heat. Add the onion, peppers and carrots and sauté for about 8 minutes, until softened.

Add the sausage meat and break it up with a spoon, then cook for 2 minutes until the sausage meat is sealed. Add the garlic, chilli powder and paprika and stir well. Add the chopped tomatoes, stock, tomato puree and Henderson's relish or Worcestershire sauce and reduce the heat slightly to a simmer. Cook for 20 minutes, stirring occasionally.

After 20 minutes, stir in the baked beans. Cook for a further 5 minutes to ensure they are thoroughly heated through. Serve!

Weekly Meal Planner

	BREAKFAST	LUNCH
MONDAY		
TUESDAY		
WEDNESDAY		
THURSDAY		
FRIDAY		
SATURDAY		
SUNDAY		

Weekly Meal Planner

DINNER	SNACK	NOTES

Day One

BREAKFAST	VALUES
TOTAL	

LUNCH	VALUES
TOTAL	

DINNER	VALUES
TOTAL	

SNACKS AND TREATS	VALUES
TOTAL	
DAILY TOTAL	

WATER

Notes

Day Two

BREAKFAST	VALUES
TOTAL	

LUNCH	VALUES
TOTAL	

DINNER	VALUES
TOTAL	

SNACKS AND TREATS	VALUES
TOTAL	
DAILY TOTAL	

WATER

○ ○ ○ ○
○ ○ ○ ○

'Keep on inspiring us to eat healthier
and cook from scratch!' **GILL**

Day Three

BREAKFAST	VALUES
TOTAL	

LUNCH	VALUES
TOTAL	

DINNER	VALUES
TOTAL	

SNACKS AND TREATS	VALUES
TOTAL	
DAILY TOTAL	

WATER

Notes

Day Four

BREAKFAST	VALUES
TOTAL	

LUNCH	VALUES
TOTAL	

DINNER	VALUES
TOTAL	

SNACKS AND TREATS	VALUES
TOTAL	
DAILY TOTAL	

WATER

○ ○ ○ ○
○ ○ ○ ○

Notes

CHICKEN, BACON *and* LEEK CRUSTLESS QUICHE

🕐 **10 MINS** | 🍲 **45 MINS** | ✕ **SERVES 8**

PER SERVING
178 KCAL / 4G CARBS

SPECIAL EQUIPMENT
24cm (9½in) quiche dish

low-calorie cooking spray
1 medium onion, peeled
    and chopped
1 medium leek, trimmed,
    washed and chopped
1 medium skinless
    chicken breast (visible
    fat removed), cut into
    1cm (½in) dice
2 smoked bacon
    medallions, cut into
    1 cm (½in) dice
1 tsp fresh thyme leaves,
    finely chopped
250g fat-free cottage
    cheese
1 tsp English mustard
    powder
6 medium eggs, beaten
    with a fork
160g reduced-fat mature
    Cheddar, finely grated
sea salt and freshly ground
    black pepper

TO ACCOMPANY *(optional)*
75g mixed salad (+ 15 kcal
    per serving)

We've packed all the flavours from our popular Chicken, Bacon and Leek Cottage Pie into a hearty, crustless quiche. It's got way more flavour and much fewer calories than a basic shop-bought quiche Lorraine! Bake the meat, veggies and creamy cheesy centre in the oven until the top is golden brown. Why not pop a portion in your lunchbox for an easy light lunch?

Everyday Light —————————————————

Preheat the oven to 180°C (fan 160°C/gas mark 4).

Spray a large frying pan with low-calorie cooking spray and place over a medium heat. Add the onion and leek and fry for 5 minutes, stirring, until starting to soften.

Add the chicken and bacon and fry, stirring, for a further 5 minutes or until the chicken is cooked through and light golden: it should not show any signs of pinkness and the juices should run clear. Stir in the thyme, remove from the heat and set aside.

Place the cottage cheese, mustard powder and 2 tablespoons of cold water in a food processor, or use a stick blender and a bowl, to blitz until smooth.

Place the eggs, cottage cheese mixture and grated Cheddar in a medium mixing bowl (or the same bowl you blended the cottage cheese in, if you used a stick blender) and stir until completely combined.

Add the cooked chicken, bacon, onion and leek mixture and season with salt and pepper. Stir to combine.

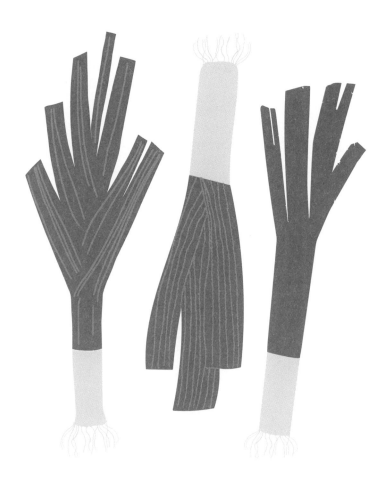

Spray the quiche dish with low-calorie cooking spray and use it to grease the dish thoroughly. Place the quiche dish on a large baking tray.

Pour the quiche mixture into the greased dish on the tray and bake in the oven for 30–35 minutes until the quiche is golden and lightly set in the centre.

Serve hot, warm or cold, with an accompaniment of your choice.

Day Five

BREAKFAST	VALUES
TOTAL	

LUNCH	VALUES
TOTAL	

DINNER	VALUES
TOTAL	

SNACKS AND TREATS	VALUES
TOTAL	
DAILY TOTAL	

WATER

○ ○ ○ ○
○ ○ ○ ○

Notes

Day Six

BREAKFAST	VALUES
TOTAL	

LUNCH	VALUES
TOTAL	

DINNER	VALUES
TOTAL	

SNACKS AND TREATS	VALUES
TOTAL	
DAILY TOTAL	

WATER

○ ○ ○ ○
○ ○ ○ ○

Notes

Day Seven

BREAKFAST	VALUES
TOTAL	

LUNCH	VALUES
TOTAL	

DINNER	VALUES
TOTAL	

SNACKS AND TREATS	VALUES
TOTAL	
DAILY TOTAL	

WATER

○ ○ ○ ○
○ ○ ○ ○

Notes

Eleven

CHANGE +/-   **CURRENT WEIGHT**

— The Week Ahead —

REMINDERS FOR THIS WEEK

LAST WEEK, THESE THINGS WENT WELL...

IN THE FREEZER   DATE   **FOOD TO USE UP**   DATE

Weekly Meal Planner

	BREAKFAST	LUNCH
MONDAY		
TUESDAY		
WEDNESDAY		
THURSDAY		
FRIDAY		
SATURDAY		
SUNDAY		

Weekly Meal Planner

DINNER	SNACK	NOTES

ITALIAN-STYLE CHICKEN PIE

⏱ **30 MINS** | 🍲 **1 HOUR 10 MINS** | ✕ **SERVES 4**

PER SERVING
419 KCAL / 48G CARBS

SPECIAL EQUIPMENT
18 x 27cm (7 x 10½in)
ovenproof dish

FOR THE FILLING
low-calorie cooking spray
250g cherry tomatoes,
    halved
2 medium onions, peeled
    and thinly sliced
2 garlic cloves, peeled and
    crushed
600g diced chicken breast
450ml chicken stock
    (1 chicken stock cube
    dissolved in 450ml
    boiling water)
¼ tsp dried oregano
100g fine green beans,
    trimmed and quartered
180g low-fat cream cheese
10g fresh basil leaves,
    stalks removed and
    leaves left whole, plus
    extra to serve
sea salt and freshly ground
    black pepper

This comforting crowd-pleasing dish is a whole meal in one pie! The chicken, green beans and roasted cherry tomatoes are simmered in a Tuscan-inspired sauce, topped with garlicky mashed potato and a sprinkle of grated Parmesan. Hearty and flavoursome, this recipe is made for batch cooking. Pop leftovers into containers and freeze for another day.

Weekly Indulgence ─────────────

Preheat the oven to 240°C (fan 220°C/gas mark 9), line a baking tray with foil and spray the foil with low-calorie cooking spray.

To make the filling, place the cherry tomato halves on the lined tray, arrange them cut side up in a single layer and spray with low-calorie cooking spray. Season with salt and pepper and roast in the oven for 15–20 minutes until they have wrinkled a little. Remove from the oven and set aside, and reduce the oven temperature to 200°C (fan 180°C/gas mark 6).

While the tomatoes are roasting, make the mashed potato for the pie topping. Place the potatoes in a large saucepan of cold water, then bring it to the boil. Reduce the heat, cover and simmer for 20 minutes until soft and tender.

Drain the potatoes well, return them to the pan, add the milk and garlic granules and mash until smooth. Season with salt and pepper. Cover and set aside while you make the pie filling.

Continue making the pie filling. Spray a large frying pan with low-calorie cooking spray and place over a medium heat. Add the onions and garlic and fry for 5 minutes until softening, then add the diced chicken and fry for 4–5 minutes to seal on all sides. Add the chicken stock and oregano and

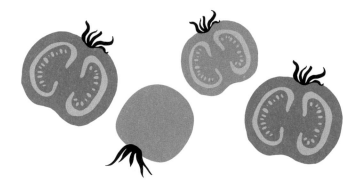

FOR THE PIE TOPPING

800g large floury potatoes, such as Maris Piper or King Edward, peeled and cut into chunks

75ml skimmed milk

1 tsp garlic granules

sea salt and freshly ground black pepper

15g Parmesan, finely grated

TO ACCOMPANY *(optional)*

80g steamed green vegetables (+ 35 kcal per serving)

stir. Partially cover with a lid or a piece of foil, then simmer for 15 minutes. Remove the lid, add the fine green beans and simmer, uncovered, for a further 5 minutes. The chicken should show no sign of pinkness and the beans should still be firm.

Remove the frying pan from the heat and stir in the cream cheese until completely blended in. If the sauce seems too thick, mix in a little water; if it seems too thin, simmer (uncovered) for a little longer to reduce the liquid.

Stir the roasted tomatoes and basil leaves, until the basil leaves are just wilting, then taste and season with salt and pepper if needed.

Place the pie filling in the ovenproof dish and spread it out evenly. Spoon the mashed potato over the pie filling and carefully spread out evenly, taking care to spread it right to the edges to seal. Use a fork to add texture to the surface of the mash.

Sprinkle the Parmesan over the top, place on a baking tray and bake in the oven for about 20 minutes until the pie is golden on top and piping hot throughout. Scatter a few fresh basil leaves on top and serve alone, or with steamed vegetables.

SWAP THIS: You could use vegetarian hard cheese, veggie stock and substitute the chicken for diced Quorn fillets if you wanted to try a meat-free version of this pie.

TIP: We've used 2 cloves of garlic in the filling and 1 teaspoon of garlic granules in the mashed potato – if you prefer a stronger garlic flavour you could add another clove or two to the filling.

Day One

BREAKFAST	VALUES
TOTAL	

LUNCH	VALUES
TOTAL	

DINNER	VALUES
TOTAL	

SNACKS AND TREATS	VALUES
TOTAL	
DAILY TOTAL	

WATER

Notes

Day Two

BREAKFAST	VALUES
TOTAL	

LUNCH	VALUES
TOTAL	

DINNER	VALUES
TOTAL	

SNACKS AND TREATS	VALUES
TOTAL	
DAILY TOTAL	

WATER

Notes

CHEESY BRAMLEY APPLE PORK

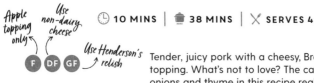

Apple topping only

Use non-dairy cheese

Use Henderson's relish

F **DF** **GF**

🕐 **10 MINS** | 🍲 **38 MINS** | ✕ **SERVES 4**

Tender, juicy pork with a cheesy, Bramley apple topping. What's not to love? The caramelised onions and thyme in this recipe really enhance the rich, meaty flavours. We love watching the cheesy topping bubble away under the grill! Serve it up with freshly steamed veggies for a filling family dinner.

PER SERVING
266 KCAL / 7.6G CARBS

low-calorie cooking spray
1 medium onion, peeled
  and thinly sliced
1 garlic clove, peeled and
  crushed
1 medium Bramley cooking
  apple (about 150g),
  peeled, cored and
  thinly sliced
2 tsp fresh thyme leaves,
  finely chopped
1 tsp Dijon mustard
1 tsp Worcestershire sauce
  or Henderson's relish
4 medium lean pork steaks
  or chops, trimmed of all
  visible fat
80g reduced-fat mature
  Cheddar, finely grated
sea salt and freshly ground
  black pepper, to taste

TO ACCOMPANY (optional)
80g steamed green
  vegetables (+ 35 kcal
  per serving)

Everyday Light

Spray a small frying pan with low-calorie cooking spray and place over a medium-low heat. Add the onion and fry for 10–15 minutes, gently and slowly, until caramelised and softened.

Add the garlic and apple to the pan of onion and stir well. Increase the heat to medium and fry for about 5 minutes until the apples are golden.

Add 60ml cold water, the thyme, mustard and Worcestershire sauce or Henderson's relish and stir.

Reduce the heat to low and cook gently for about 5 minutes until the apples have broken down into a soft mash. You may need to add a tablespoon or two of water if the mixture starts to dry out – the mixture should have a thick, spreadable consistency. Season to taste with salt and pepper. Set aside.

Preheat the grill to high. Spray a baking tray with low-calorie cooking spray. Season the pork steaks or chops with a little salt and pepper and place on the baking tray. Place the tray of pork under the grill for about 8 minutes, turning the steaks or chops occasionally, until cooked through and there's no sign of pinkness. They may need less or more time under the grill, depending on their thickness.

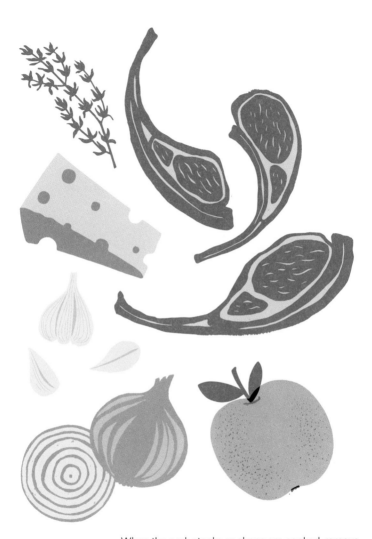

SWAP THIS:
If you prefer, swap the
fresh thyme for fresh
sage, a herb that works
equally well with pork.

When the pork steaks or chops are cooked, remove
them from the grill and reduce the temperature to
medium. Spread the apple mixture evenly on top of
the pork, sprinkle the cheese on top of the apple
mixture and place under the grill for 5 minutes until
the cheese has melted and is golden. Serve at once
with an accompaniment of your choice.

171

Day Three

BREAKFAST	VALUES
TOTAL	

LUNCH	VALUES
TOTAL	

DINNER	VALUES
TOTAL	

SNACKS AND TREATS	VALUES
TOTAL	
DAILY TOTAL	

WATER

○ ○ ○ ○
○ ○ ○ ○

Notes

WEEK 11

Day Four

BREAKFAST	VALUES
TOTAL	

LUNCH	VALUES
TOTAL	

DINNER	VALUES
TOTAL	

SNACKS AND TREATS	VALUES
TOTAL	
DAILY TOTAL	

WATER

○○○○
○○○○

Notes

Day Five

BREAKFAST	VALUES
TOTAL	

LUNCH	VALUES
TOTAL	

DINNER	VALUES
TOTAL	

SNACKS AND TREATS	VALUES
TOTAL	
DAILY TOTAL	

WATER

○ ○ ○ ○
○ ○ ○ ○

Notes

Day Six

BREAKFAST	VALUES
TOTAL	

LUNCH	VALUES
TOTAL	

DINNER	VALUES
TOTAL	

SNACKS AND TREATS	VALUES
TOTAL	
DAILY TOTAL	

WATER

⬡ ⬡ ⬡ ⬡
⬡ ⬡ ⬡ ⬡

'Just received my new food planner!
So pretty and will hopefully keep me on
track with my healthy eating!' **DARCIE**

Day Seven

BREAKFAST	VALUES
TOTAL	

LUNCH	VALUES
TOTAL	

DINNER	VALUES
TOTAL	

SNACKS AND TREATS	VALUES
TOTAL	
DAILY TOTAL	

WATER

Notes

Shopping List 1

....
....
....
....
....
....
....
....
....
....
....
....
....
....
....
....
....
....
....

Shopping List 2

....
....
....
....
....
....
....
....
....
....
....
....
....
....
....
....
....
....

Shopping List 1

....
....
....
....
....
....
....
....
....
....
....
....
....
....
....
....
....
....

Shopping List 2

....
....
....
....
....
....
....
....
....
....
....
....
....
....
....
....
....
....

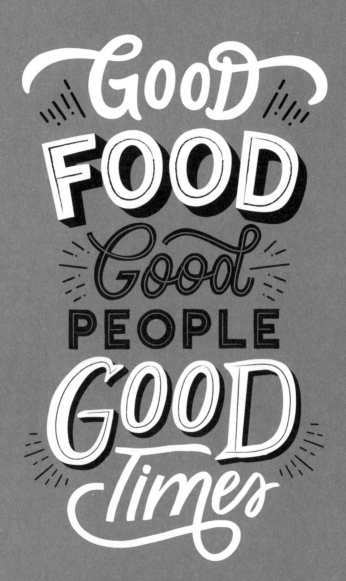

Twelve

CHANGE +/-   **CURRENT WEIGHT**

The Week Ahead

REMINDERS FOR THIS WEEK

LAST WEEK, THESE THINGS WENT WELL...

IN THE FREEZER   DATE   **FOOD TO USE UP**   DATE

GREEK-STYLE
LEEKS *and* RICE

Use reduced-fat
Greek-style
salad cheese
 Use GF
stock cubes

(V) (F) (BF) (GF)

🕐 **5 MINS** | 🍲 **35 MINS** | ✕ **SERVES 4**

PER SERVING
264 KCAL / 44G CARBS

low-calorie cooking spray
2 leeks, trimmed, rinsed
    and thinly sliced
1 onion, peeled and diced
2 garlic cloves, peeled and
    crushed
200g Arborio or risotto rice
900ml vegetable stock
    (2 vegetable stock cubes
    dissolved in 900ml
    boiling water)
juice of 1 lemon
100g reduced-fat feta
    cheese, crumbled
handful of fresh dill,
    chopped
freshly ground black
    pepper

TO ACCOMPANY *(optional)*
75g mixed salad (+ 15 kcal
    per serving)

A little like a risotto, this dish is our slimming-friendly take on a popular Greek recipe, Spanakorizo. You only need a handful of ingredients and 40 minutes to throw this together, so it's ideal for a midweek dinner. The leeks cook slowly until they're lovely and sweet – the flavour contrasts so well with the salty feta cheese. We love the leftovers for lunch!

Everyday Light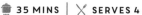

Spray a large saucepan with low-calorie cooking spray and place over a low heat. Add the leeks and onion and sauté for 15 minutes. Don't rush this. The long, slow cooking of the leeks brings out the sweet flavours that are essential for this dish. You don't have to stand over the pan, just stir every couple of minutes to ensure they cook evenly and don't stick.

Add the garlic and cook for another minute, then add the rice and stir well. Pour in the stock, increase the heat and bring to the boil, then reduce the heat to low and cook for 20 minutes, stirring occasionally, until the rice is tender and most of the liquid has been absorbed. Remove from the heat.

Stir in the lemon juice and the feta, dill and a good pinch of pepper. Cover with a lid and allow to stand for 5 minutes before serving.

Weekly Meal Planner

	BREAKFAST	LUNCH
MONDAY		
TUESDAY		
WEDNESDAY		
THURSDAY		
FRIDAY		
SATURDAY		
SUNDAY		

Weekly Meal Planner

DINNER	SNACK	NOTES

Day One

BREAKFAST	VALUES
TOTAL	

LUNCH	VALUES
TOTAL	

DINNER	VALUES
TOTAL	

SNACKS AND TREATS	VALUES
TOTAL	
DAILY TOTAL	

WATER

◊ ◊ ◊ ◊
◊ ◊ ◊ ◊

Notes

Day Two

BREAKFAST	VALUES
TOTAL	

LUNCH	VALUES
TOTAL	

DINNER	VALUES
TOTAL	

SNACKS AND TREATS	VALUES
TOTAL	
DAILY TOTAL	

WATER

○ ○ ○ ○
○ ○ ○ ○

'With a busy family who all love your recipes, this planner will be a valued addition to my PON collection.' **HELEN**

Day Three

BREAKFAST	VALUES
TOTAL	

LUNCH	VALUES
TOTAL	

DINNER	VALUES
TOTAL	

SNACKS AND TREATS	VALUES
TOTAL	
DAILY TOTAL	

WATER

○ ○ ○ ○
○ ○ ○ ○

Notes

Day Four

BREAKFAST	VALUES
TOTAL	

LUNCH	VALUES
TOTAL	

DINNER	VALUES
TOTAL	

SNACKS AND TREATS	VALUES
TOTAL	
DAILY TOTAL	

WATER

○ ○ ○ ○
○ ○ ○ ○

Notes

BEEF *and* SPRING ONION CHOW MEIN

🕐 **10 MINS*** | 🍲 **15 MINS** | ✕ **SERVES 4**

*10 MINS, PLUS 30 MINS MARINATING

(F) (BF) (DF)

PER SERVING
394 KCAL / 52G CARBS

400g lean beef stir-fry strips
4 x 50g nests of dried egg
    noodles
low-calorie cooking spray
2 large garlic cloves, peeled
    and finely chopped
2cm (¾in) piece of root
    ginger, peeled and
    finely chopped
1 large onion, peeled
    and sliced
1 medium red pepper,
    deseeded and sliced
    into strips
6 spring onions, trimmed
    and cut into 5cm (2in)
    lengths
3 tbsp dark soy sauce
2 tbsp oyster sauce
2 tbsp rice vinegar
1 tsp granulated sweetener
2 small pak choi (about
    100g each), cut into
    4cm (1½in) pieces
100g fresh beansprouts

Inspired by the flavours of one of our favourite
takeaway meals, this Beef and Spring Onion
Chow Mein has been an instant hit in our house.
Super quick to stir fry, it's a family-friendly choice
for Fakeaway night, packed with fresh veggies,
tender strips of beef and filling egg noodles. You
can even batch cook this and freeze or chill the
leftovers for another day.

Everyday Light ─────────────────────

First, marinade the beef. Place the beef strips in
a medium bowl. Add the cornflour, soy sauce,
sweetener, salt and Chinese 5-spice. Using clean
hands, mix thoroughly until the beef is evenly
coated. Cover and set aside to marinate for
30 minutes.

While the beef is marinating, cook the noodles in
a medium saucepan of boiling water according to
the packet instructions. Drain, then rinse the cooked
noodles under cold running water and set aside.

Spray a large frying pan or wok with low-calorie
cooking spray and place over a medium-high heat.
When it's really hot, add the marinated beef and
stir-fry for 2 minutes to seal and lightly brown.

Add the garlic and ginger to the pan or wok and
stir-fry for a further 1–2 minutes, taking care not to
burn the garlic. Increase the heat to high, add the
onion, red pepper and spring onion and stir-fry for
3 minutes, then add the soy sauce, oyster sauce,
rice vinegar and sweetener and stir well. Stir in the
cooked noodles, pak choi and beansprouts and
stir-fry for 1–2 minutes, taking care not to overcook
the vegetables.

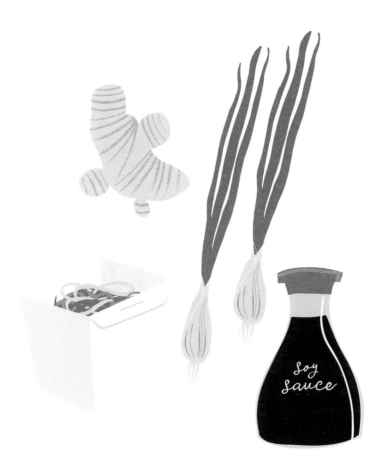

FOR THE MARINADE
1 tbsp cornflour
2 tbsp dark soy sauce
1 tsp granulated sweetener
½ tsp salt
small pinch of Chinese
  5-spice

The vegetables should still retain some crispness and be lightly coated with the soy and oyster sauces.

Serve at once.

TIPS: It's important to be organised before starting this recipe. Prepare all the ingredients before you start and put them in small bowls so that you're ready when you need to add them to the frying pan or wok. If you're still cutting up vegetables while stir-frying, it's likely you'll end up overcooking the stir fry. You need the pan or wok to be really hot and you need to keep the ingredients moving around the pan while they fry: this helps keep them tasting fresh and will retain some crispness. Cut the vegetables uniformly to help ensure even cooking.

Day Five

BREAKFAST	VALUES
TOTAL	

LUNCH	VALUES
TOTAL	

DINNER	VALUES
TOTAL	

SNACKS AND TREATS	VALUES
TOTAL	
DAILY TOTAL	

WATER

○ ○ ○ ○
○ ○ ○ ○

Notes

Day Six

BREAKFAST	VALUES
TOTAL	

LUNCH	VALUES
TOTAL	

DINNER	VALUES
TOTAL	

SNACKS AND TREATS	VALUES
TOTAL	
DAILY TOTAL	

WATER

○ ○ ○ ○
○ ○ ○ ○

Notes

Day Seven

BREAKFAST	VALUES
TOTAL	

LUNCH	VALUES
TOTAL	

DINNER	VALUES
TOTAL	

SNACKS AND TREATS	VALUES
TOTAL	
DAILY TOTAL	

WATER

◊ ◊ ◊ ◊
◊ ◊ ◊ ◊

Notes

Thirteen

CHANGE +/-   **CURRENT WEIGHT**

— The Week Ahead ————————————

REMINDERS FOR THIS WEEK

LAST WEEK, THESE THINGS WENT WELL...

IN THE FREEZER   DATE   **FOOD TO USE UP**   DATE

SWEET *and* SOUR HALLOUMI

   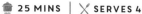

PER SERVING
298 KCAL / 33G CARBS

low-calorie cooking spray
1 x 225g pack reduced-fat halloumi, cut into 2cm (¾in) cubes
1 medium onion, peeled and sliced
2 mixed peppers, deseeded and sliced
2 garlic cloves, peeled and crushed
2cm (¾in) piece of root ginger, peeled and grated
350ml vegetable stock (1 vegetable stock cube dissolved in 350ml boiling water)
100g tomato puree
1 x 225g tin pineapple chunks in juice, drained and juice reserved
3 tbsp rice vinegar
1 tbsp light soy sauce
3 tbsp brown granulated sweetener (you can use white sweetener or brown sugar if you prefer)
1 x 200g tin water chestnuts, drained

TO ACCOMPANY *(optional)*
50g raw basmati rice per portion, cooked according to packet instructions (+ 173 kcal per 125g cooked serving)

We love the sticky goodness of a sweet and sour dish from the takeaway. Our Sweet and Sour Halloumi recipe recreates those flavours without all the calories. We've used firm yet gooey halloumi as the base of our dish, combined with the refreshing sweetness of juicy pineapple chunks. It's the whole family's new favourite Fakeaway!

Everyday Light ——————————————

Spray a large non-stick wok or frying pan with low-calorie cooking spray and place over a high heat. Add the halloumi and cook for 2–3 minutes, gently stirring until it is well browned. Remove from the pan and put to one side.

Reduce the heat to medium, wipe out the wok or pan and give it another spray with low-calorie cooking spray. Add the onion and peppers and stir-fry for 5 minutes. Add the garlic and ginger and cook for a further minute.

Whisk together the stock, tomato puree, reserved pineapple juice, rice vinegar, soy sauce and sweetener in a bowl, then add to the wok or pan. Bring to the boil then adjust the heat to a simmer and cook for 10 minutes.

After 10 minutes, add the pineapple chunks, water chestnuts and browned halloumi to the pan, stir well and cook for a further 5 minutes until everything is thoroughly heated through. Serve!

Day One

BREAKFAST	VALUES
TOTAL	

LUNCH	VALUES
TOTAL	

DINNER	VALUES
TOTAL	

SNACKS AND TREATS	VALUES
TOTAL	
DAILY TOTAL	

WATER

○ ○ ○ ○
○ ○ ○ ○

Notes

Weekly Meal Planner

	BREAKFAST	LUNCH
MONDAY		
TUESDAY		
WEDNESDAY		
THURSDAY		
FRIDAY		
SATURDAY		
SUNDAY		

Weekly Meal Planner

DINNER	SNACK	NOTES

Day Two

BREAKFAST	VALUES
TOTAL	

LUNCH	VALUES
TOTAL	

DINNER	VALUES
TOTAL	

SNACKS AND TREATS	VALUES
TOTAL	
DAILY TOTAL	

WATER

○ ○ ○ ○
○ ○ ○ ○

Notes

Day Three

BREAKFAST	VALUES
TOTAL	

LUNCH	VALUES
TOTAL	

DINNER	VALUES
TOTAL	

SNACKS AND TREATS	VALUES
TOTAL	
DAILY TOTAL	

WATER

○ ○ ○ ○

○ ○ ○ ○

Notes

Day Four

BREAKFAST	VALUES
TOTAL	

LUNCH	VALUES
TOTAL	

DINNER	VALUES
TOTAL	

SNACKS AND TREATS	VALUES
TOTAL	
DAILY TOTAL	

WATER

○ ○ ○ ○
○ ○ ○ ○

Notes

Day Five

BREAKFAST	VALUES
TOTAL	

LUNCH	VALUES
TOTAL	

DINNER	VALUES
TOTAL	

SNACKS AND TREATS	VALUES
TOTAL	
DAILY TOTAL	

WATER

Notes

Day Six

BREAKFAST	VALUES
TOTAL	

LUNCH	VALUES
TOTAL	

DINNER	VALUES
TOTAL	

SNACKS AND TREATS	VALUES
TOTAL	
DAILY TOTAL	

WATER

◇ ◇ ◇ ◇
◇ ◇ ◇ ◇

Notes

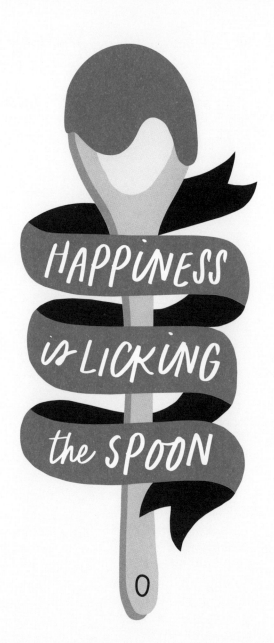

Shopping List 1

....

....

....

....

....

....

....

....

....

....

....

....

....

....

....

....

....

....

....

Shopping List 2

....

....

....

....

....

....

....

....

....

....

....

....

....

....

....

....

....

....

....

Day Seven

BREAKFAST	VALUES
TOTAL	

LUNCH	VALUES
TOTAL	

DINNER	VALUES
TOTAL	

SNACKS AND TREATS	VALUES
TOTAL	
DAILY TOTAL	

WATER

○ ○ ○ ○
○ ○ ○ ○

Notes

Index

Acknowledgements

We want to say a huge thank you to all of our followers on social media and all those who make our recipes. Without you, this planner and everything else we do just wouldn't be possible.

Thank you to our publisher Carole Tonkinson, Martha Burley, Zainab Dawood, Jodie Mullish, Jess Duffy, Sian Gardiner, Holly Martin, Mel Four, Sarah Badhan and the rest of the team at Bluebird and Pan Macmillan. You've been such an inspiration and we couldn't do this without you. Thank you for helping us make this happen. Massive thanks also to our agent Clare Hulton for your unwavering support and guidance.

Thanks to everyone at Nic&Lou, especially to Emma Wells. You always take our ideas and bring them to life in the most fantastic way.

Special thanks go to Sophie Fryer, Katie Mitchell, Lisa Allinson, Cate Meadows, Sharon Fitzpatrick, Holly Levell, Hannah Cutting, Ellie Drinkwater, Laura Valentine and Nick Nicolaou – thanks for all your hard work during the making of this planner. Additional thanks go to Matthew Maney, Rubi Bourne, Vince Bourne and Cheryl Lloyd, Jacob Lathbury and Jessica Molyneux – thank you for your support. We're so proud to work with you guys x

No acknowledgement would be complete without a mention for our various furry babies – Mildred, Brandi, Ginger Cat and Freda.

Laura Davis *Acknowledgements*

Thanks to Helen Davis, Steve Davis, Jennie Darke, Nick Darke, Isla Darke and Millie Darke and all of the Spence clan for your constant love. For Elsie & Geoff Spence who gave us all the world.

Kate & Kay Allinson *Acknowledgements*

With thanks, as ever, to Paul Allinson – none of this would ever have been possible without yours and Cath's support. Everything we do will always be for Cath x